THE PSYCHOLOGY OF ANIMALS IN RELATION TO HUMAN PSYCHOLOGY

T0174037

Founded by C. K. Ogden

The International Library of Psychology

COMPARATIVE PSYCHOLOGY
In 4 Volumes

THE PSYCHOLOGY OF ANIMALS IN RELATION TO HUMAN PSYCHOLOGY

F ALVERDES

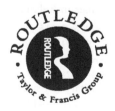

First published in 1932
by Routledge, Trench, Trubner & Co., Ltd.

Reprinted in 1999, 2000
by Routledge
2 Park Square, Milton Park, Abingdon, Oxfordshire OX14 4RN

711 Third Avenue, New York, NY 10017
First issued in paperback 2014

Routledge is an imprint of the Taylor and Francis Group,
an informa company

Transferred to Digital Printing 2007

All rights reserved. No part of this book may be reprinted or reproduced
or utilized in any form or by any electronic, mechanical, or other means,
now known or hereafter invented, including photocopying
and recording, or in any information storage or retrieval system, without
permission in writing from the publishers.

The publishers have made every effort to contact authors/copyright holders
of the works reprinted in the *International Library of Psychology*.
This has not been possible in every case, however, and we would
welcome correspondence from those individuals/companies
we have been unable to trace.

These reprints are taken from original copies of each book. In many cases
the condition of these originals is not perfect. The publisher has gone to
great lengths to ensure the quality of these reprints, but wishes to point
out that certain characteristics of the original copies will, of necessity, be
apparent in reprints thereof.

British Library Cataloguing in Publication Data
A CIP catalogue record for this book
is available from the British Library

The Psychology of Animals in Relation to Human Psychology
ISBN 978-0-415-20977-9 (hbk)
ISBN 978-0-415-75791-1 (pbk)
Comparative Psychology: 4 Volumes
ISBN 978-0-415-21127-7
The International Library of Psychology: 204 Volumes
ISBN 978-0-415-19132-6

CONTENTS

INTRODUCTION

THE man of science is not infrequently accused of devoting too much attention to details, and so losing sight of broad generalities in a maze of single facts. It is sometimes said that the learned have neither the power, nor even the desire, to make the subjects they have chosen for their life-work accessible to a wider public. Often enough, it is maintained, these subjects are not suitable to such popularization, since they are too remote and specialized.

We shall not here consider to what extent such reproaches are justified. But we may at least remember that exceptions exist. In the following pages I offer my own attempt at a short description of such parts of animal psychology as are of interest to a wider public, at the same time exhibiting the many and various relations existing between human and animal psychology. Animal Psychology is a branch of science which has already developed a complicated technical vocabulary—of necessity, since without it the observations could not be properly described, and a common understanding between individual workers would be impossible. In the present connection I shall, however, avoid as far as possible the use of technical terms. And as in the case of many other branches of research, a person not acquainted with animal psychology would regard many lines of investigation as entirely beside the point and superfluous, if he heard of them apart from their connections. Only these connections give to an apparently trifling detail its meaning and importance.

It is not my intention to add one more to the existing full accounts of animal psychology. My wish is rather to describe in popular language such parts of the subject as appear to me to be of most importance today; and at the same time I hope, by setting out from a more general biological point of view, to be able to give some new suggestions regarding human psychology. The purpose of the book led of itself to the necessity for avoiding too many details, and confining myself to the selection of those points most interesting to a general audience.

[Systematic names of organisms are italicised only on their first appearance, in the belief that the general reader will find this more agreeable than the persistence in italics usual in English scientific works.—H.S.H.]

The Psychology of Animals
In Relation to Human Psychology

CHAPTER I

Difference between living and non-living nature.—The " End "
(aim, object, purpose, goal) and the " Whole " as biological
fictions.—" The End determines the Means ", and " the
Whole determines the Parts ".

OF all the branches of learning which make up the science
of zoology, that of Animal Psychology appears to me
personally to be the highest. Anyone who has worked
through all the various departments of zoology, through
the study of various animal forms, through morphology,
embryology, theory of descent, comparative physiology,
and all the rest of the many branches, should, I think,
find at last in Animal Psychology the most important
teaching of all, and one of particular value as regards
a deeper view of man and his place in Nature. My object
in this book is to introduce the reader to the chief problems
of Animal Psychology—or more cautiously speaking,
those problems which appear to me personally as out-
standing, and of most immediate interest.

Since this book is addressed to the lay reader, no special
knowledge of the subject will be assumed, and only
matters of general interest will be selected for discussion.

By way of introduction, it is necessary to deal with

A   I

some preliminary questions which may seem to the reader
rather remote from the subject. The first of these is the
general question of the nature of life.

Life is bound up with matter, but we are unable to
say what it really is. We can only state what are the
properties which characterize living organisms, and how
these creatures differ from non-living nature. We are
then confronted with the problem of what agency maintains all the phenomena of life in continued activity.

Most readers will have heard of the battle between
Mechanism and *Vitalism*, at least as far as the terms
themselves go. Mechanism proposes to explain life
phenomena as the interaction of highly complicated
physico-chemical processes, which take place in the
substances constituting the organism. Vitalism, on the
other hand, assumes that matter alone can never give
rise to the phenomena of life, but that an immaterial
agent must be present, which has power over non-living
matter; this agent is supposed to interfere with, and
regulate continuously, the chemical and physical processes, in order that a living organism may come into
being and continue to exist. Generally speaking, this
agent is regarded as more or less analogous with the
conscious human psyche. In my opinion, this conflict
between mechanism and vitalism is fundamentally impossible to settle. It is beyond the powers of our human
mind to decide whether life processes take place solely
in accordance with physico-chemical laws, or whether a
special agent is behind them and controls them. In this
matter, therefore, we must be modest: and in this case
—as also in others—it is better to recognize clearly the

limits of our knowledge and insight, than to conceal our ignorance under mere words.

If we consider non-living nature, we see that it is in a state of balance or equilibrium : and when a disturbance occurs, the corresponding restoration of equilibrium takes place at once. The same is true of the single living being ; normally, the various functions of its body are in harmony with itself and with the external world, and when this harmony is upset, a new state of balance is soon set up. But there is a fundamental difference between the processes which lead to a balance on the one hand in the non-living, and on the other in the living world : in the latter, they ensure the preservation of the living organism *as such*, its continuation as an individual, as a whole complete in all its parts. They are such as to ensure both its persistence and its integrity. There is nothing of this kind in non-living nature ; the heavenly bodies, the continents, mountain ranges, masses of rock, rivers, are never organisms akin to living things, and hence are not capable of self-regulation, as are the latter.

We will here introduce a fiction. We say that the insurance of persistence and integrity is the " biological purpose " of the regulatory processes taking place in the organism. But when we make use of this idea, we must be perfectly clear that we are dealing with something which we are putting into nature. Experience has taught us for example, that when one organ is lost, another can function so as to compensate for the loss ; if a human being loses one kidney the other enlarges and thus is able to do alone the work which was originally done by the two. In this and similar cases, we assume that it is the purpose, object, or aim of the processes we observe to secure the organism against death and dissolution, to maintain it as a complete whole, as an individual. In non-living events, on the other hand, we are never able to discover such a meaning or aim ; we must therefore say that these processes are apart from all aim or meaning, not aimless or meaningless, since this can only be said in cases where the meaningful also exists.

I would like at this point to meet an objection which can perhaps be made against the notion of an imaginary purpose in the biological sense. I said before, and repeat here, that we deduce this purpose from experience. When in a large number of cases and in given circumstances the same result is always obtained when, for example, we cut one leg off each of 100 newts and the loss is made good in all cases, we regard the reconstitution of the complete animal as the aim and object of the processes of growth which take place. We are dealing in statistics, so to speak, and they teach us in this instance, that in 100 per cent of cases of a certain operation, to wit the cutting off of a leg, the same effect occurs, namely, that it grows again. It may now be said that in inorganic nature also, statistics lead to the same result ; that like causes produce like effects. We might, for example, allow 100 balls to roll down a hill, and all of them would come to rest at the same spot in the valley. Are we then, it may be asked, to describe this spot as the " aim " or " object " of the balls ? To say the least, this would be to weaken very greatly the idea of purpose which we have just set up.

The difference becomes plain when we vary the conditions of the experiments which we make on living and non-living objects. Thus we may carry out our experiments on the newts by treating each one of them differently as regards the way we cut the leg, never completely removing it, but leaving in every case more or less of it ; here again the result of the process of regeneration is the restoration of a complete leg. Or we may cut a fresh-water polyp (*Hydra*) or a worm into numerous pieces ; every single piece replaces what is missing, and so becomes a complete animal. In the latter case it is noteworthy that every single part is different from every other, not only, it may be, as regards size, but above all because each part is derived from a different part of the original body. All of them, therefore, must attain their aim of the restoration of the complete animal by different means. This leads us to an important law which holds for biological processes : " the end determines the means ".

But may not this law perhaps be applied to the processes taking place in the inorganic world ? Let us return to our 100 balls, which we will again allow to roll downhill. But we will now no longer choose the old path, but allow one ball to roll down at one point, another at another, with the result that none reaches the original goal. This is a proof that in the first experiment with the balls, though all of them reached the same place, this place was not the aim or object of the balls, in the biological sense.

Obviously, our law that " the end determines the means " is nothing more than a fiction ; it has merely to describe relationships which we recognize as such.

We will now consider how widely this law holds. Does
it hold only for the processes of regeneration which we
have been considering ?   Let us observe a series of repre-
sentatives of various species of animals, as regards their
behaviour when endeavouring to reach a certain object,
a source of attraction.   A bird, for example, towards
which we throw a piece of food, may hasten to it by
flying or running, or even by a mixture of the two ; and
if we are dealing with a water-bird, a third possibility
exists, namely swimming.   The three modes of locomotion
which we have named, running, flying, swimming, depend
upon entirely different kinds of muscular activity ; and
if flying is combined with running or swimming, we
have again something quite different from running or
swimming alone.   The birds are thus able to approach the
food in all kinds of ways, they make use of various
" means " ; but what the bird actually does is determined
by the single fact, that it is striving to reach its aim.
The same is true of a winged insect, to which we offer
a source of light in a darkened room ;   it may approach
it running or flying.   In the same way, a water insect,
which we observe in an aquarium, may strive to reach
a certain goal either by running on the bottom, or
swimming.

The majority of animals run in the direction of the
long axis of their bodies, but an animal is able, on occasion,
to move sideways or at right angles, if its ends are served
thereby.   Here also the means are varied in accordance
with the end.   In the case of certain crustacea, for example
the common crab (*Carcinus*) or the hermit crab (*Eupagurus*)
we see, by way of contrast to other animals, that move-

ment in the direction of the body axis is rarer; they more frequently move sideways or diagonally, and move more rapidly thus. What is important in this connection is this: in the course of a single journey undertaken by the animal for the purpose of reaching a certain goal, it may continually change the direction in which its body points with reference to its path from straight ahead to any angle to right or left, without the straightness of the path being influenced in any way. But every time that a new orientation is assumed, the muscles of the legs have to act somewhat differently; here again it is the " end " which determines the " means " chosen.

Let us consider our own walking, or that of any animal, such as a beetle. If a man or a beetle commences to take a step, the goal of the movement thus begun is the completion of the step. And according to the nature of the external situation as it is met with, that is, according to the nature of the ground, the means used to attain this end are varied. This end is not, of course, assumed to be a " consciously grasped objective ", but simply the object which we regard as determining a biological movement which we observe. (We shall deal with the problem of consciousness in the next chapter.)

Higher animals, apes for example, are capable of attaining an end by roundabout ways. We attach to the roof of a large cage a fruit of some kind. The chimpanzee, for example, is able to make use of various possibilities for gaining possession of the fruit. He may run to the wall of the cage, and climb up it and along the roof, and so reach the fruit. If the roof offers no holds to enable him to traverse it, he may fetch a stick and strike at the fruit until it falls down. W. Koehler and Bierens de Haan have further shown that apes will fetch boxes and pile them one upon the other, in order so to reach the fruit. Each of the various actions we have described may be further subdivided into parts. We then see that running to the side of the cage, or to fetch a stick or boxes, are actions which in themselves do not bring the apes nearer to the object, but rather first of all take them away from it. Regarded simply, these actions appear meaningless, and only the serial arrangement of the actions in accordance with the situation gives sense to the resulting total action. We are thus presented with the possibility of varying our fictional rule concerning the end and the means as follows : " the whole determines the parts ".

We may then perform an experiment by making it impossible for an experimental animal to use its ordinary means of progression : in the case of animals possessing a considerable number of limbs, we may, for example, amputate several. Take the common crab (*Carcinus*), which possesses eight legs. We can remove from our experimental crabs a number of these legs wholly or partially and in various combinations, but the animals always retain the power, even in extreme cases of disablement, of making straight for a desired point.

Let us consider a highly complicated activity of a quite special kind, the construction of its web by the spider. Every species constructs a special form of web characteristic of it, but in the single cases the external conditions are never exactly similar ; for the animal may at one time spin its web in a four-cornered hole in a wall, for example, at another between two beams meeting at right-angles, at another between two bushes, and so on. In each case it is necessary to attach the first threads in a different manner; but what then appears is always the style of web peculiar to the species. Here again, therefore, it is the end that determines the means, and the whole that determines the parts. If we injure such a web not too seriously, the spider very soon repairs the damage. This process also fits in with our fictional rules.

In my remarks concerning our fiction of the aim or end of biological action, I started from regeneration; I then extended the notion to various actions and activities of animals. It can now be shown to hold for the whole of biological happening. A further example will illustrate this. When we study in the case of an animal the embryonic and larval development up to the reproductive stage, we are confronted with a series of what are often quite different stages. We then may introduce the fiction: the adult individual is the end, the various stages of development are the means: or we may also state the matter thus: the total development is the "whole", the single stages are the "parts". K. E. von Baer, over a hundred years ago, compared the development of the individual with a melody. In the latter, as we know, the sounds are not strung together anyhow; a relation exists between the first and the last note, in such a way that not merely does the first influence the last, but also the last the first. The whole melody is the end, the various notes are the means; or the melody is the whole, the notes are the parts.

However, what is the nature of a melody ? Is it perhaps

something that belongs to non-living nature ? If the latter were the case, would it not lead to the conclusion that many phenomena in inorganic nature are similar to embryonic development ? Now, a melody is not an " inorganic event ", but is produced by its creator—a living human being—on the basis of a conception of the whole which he forms, and which is the occasion of this melody arising in his mind ; it is reproduced from time to time by other living creatures, the performers ; it only exists at all when a living creature, a human being, creates it and recreates it.

CHAPTER II

General remarks on scientific statement, and more concerning
the fictional mode of regarding biological facts.—Consciousness, freedom of will, psyche.

IN the last chapter we started from the difference between
living and non-living natural bodies. I said that it was
fundamentally impossible to decide whether the course
of life processes results only from chemical and physical
phenomena, or whether there is behind them a special
non-material, psyche-like agent. In order to make the
difference between the living and the non-living particularly clear, I introduced some fictions, which were
to be applied only to biology. I spoke of the wholeness
of the individual, of the maintenance of a whole as the
end and object of biological processes ; this end is attained
by living creatures by means which differ from case to
case. We finally arrived at the following two rules ;
" the end determines the means " and " the whole determines the parts ". In the application of these two
fictional sentences to biological events, we see the much
debated " self-rule of life ".

It is possible that the whole way in which I have
presented and expressed the matter has aroused your
strong opposition. You are perhaps of the opinion that
the scientist—and therefore also the biologist—should
deal only with what is really given, whereas I have
repeatedly spoken to you of fiction. For this reason it

would be well for us to come to an understanding concerning the nature of scientific investigation and of the description of scientific observation. Such a description can only take place by that being emphasized which appears important to the observer. Accordingly, experience teaches us that in matters of daily life two observers may find quite different things of importance, and hence give two completely different descriptions of the same event. Even one and the same person may take a completely different view of identical events, according to his experience just previous to their observation. Regarded in this way, the tendency, for example, towards mechanistic or vitalistic viewpoint is chiefly a question of personal necessity determined from within ; in one's inmost heart one desires the world to be constituted thus or thus, and seizes upon the necessary " proofs " to form a foundation for one's view. And if in the case of a given person the nature of his world-view changes in course of time, those " proofs " which had hitherto been rejected will suddenly appear important, and " directly convincing ".

But what quite generally is the way in which our conscious ego places itself in relationship with the external world ? It is our sense organs alone which are the means of this contact. All that we observe goes through the filter of our sense organs, and what cannot pass through these does not " exist " for us at all. The data received by our sense organs are conveyed to our central nervous system. This may be from time to time in very different conditions. For we are not even the same from one moment to the next. In other words, the sense data which we receive may meet from case to case a central nervous system of quite different character, and prepared in quite a different way, and hence they may be made use of in quite a different manner. But the mosaic of sense data will always be worked up in our " thinking organ " into whole perceptions ; what is mirrored there is in the form of whole pictures ; and it is from this complete picture that we derive the abstractions and fictions that we need to comprehend and reproduce the external event with which we have been in contact. Let us be clear about the matter : we never come directly into contact with external things " as they really are ". For what is there in us that " really knows ", and is able to get into direct contact with " the things outside " ?

In view of the constitution of our human thinking apparatus, there is no other means left to us than that of working with whole abstractions. The fact that concepts such as " the animal ", " the insect ", are pure abstractions, everyone will agree ; but even when I describe a particular individual beetle as " this beetle " I thereby make a statement concerning a wholeness relationship grasped by me as such ; for the expression " this beetle " is already an abstraction, derived from the simultaneous observation of a large number of details of this animal's body. When I say " this beetle is running ", this is correspondingly the integrated sum of a large number of single processes.

Our manner of thus grasping wholes is unconnected with our voluntary and conscious intention ; it cannot be rationally explained as regards its origin, its nature, and its laws ; it is for us something primarily given. We are only in a position to determine by observation and experiment the statistical rules according to which it takes place.

This immediately raises the question as to how far life altogether is rational, that is to say, capable of being comprehended by our intellect. We will proceed to extend at once the problem thus raised, by linking it with the question as to what extent not only life, but also the whole of natural events, are capable of being rationally understood. I will state shortly where the limits lie, or rather, where they appear to me to lie. We have already seen that " knowledge " depends much less upon the object to be known than upon the subject which knows it. Hence it is a matter of the mental structure of the observer, whether he emphasizes and regards as important what is comprehensible by the intellect, or what is irrational, in life and in world events generally. If we attempt to account to ourselves concerning the origin of life, or of the world itself, and how it happens that everything is just as it is, and is happening as it is and not otherwise, there remains for us nothing to do but to admit " we do not know and we never shall know ". For everything connected with these questions is irrational. People of course exist for whom the facts of life and of the world appear self-evident, and who are entirely insensitive to the problematical nature of the world and life. Whoever is willing to limit himself in this way, and feels completely satisfied when he has discovered the laws according to which observed events take place, may well arrive at the view that the world can be explained purely rationally. As opposed to this, we may express our own view by the following image :

all that is possible for us is to determine, as regards the course of the world, the rules of the game, so to speak ; but the origin of the game itself and of its rules, to keep the metaphor, is completely beyond our knowledge. I regard it as necessary to emphasize this, since even at the present time, natural science is continually called upon as chief witness to testify in favour of the purely mechanistic world view. An historical " explanation ", that is to say, an " explanation " from what has happened hitherto, is merely an apparent explanation ; for even if we are able to state in what way anything has become what it is and as we see it today, this tells us nothing whatever concerning its origin, and for what reason it has become what it is. We may therefore say that it is waste of time to search for the origin of life ; and the question of the " meaning " or " object " of life becomes —at any rate in the light of our present point of view— a merely apparent problem, for meaning and object were only fictions for us. As the fictional end of numerous life phenomena at least, we assumed the maintenance of a whole—but this whole itself was only a fiction. Of course, not each and every biological process is to be regarded as having for its object the maintenance of a whole ; for there are others which have the opposite effect, for example all which lead to disease and death. And along with these, there may well be many which are indifferent as regards the whole. Furthermore, we also find in organisms, processes and body parts which in so far point beyond the individual being, as they allow us to conceive an imagined whole transcending the individual. These are the processes and organs which are connected with reproduction, with the care of off-spring, and with other relationships to the species as a whole; and we may then sometimes find it useful to regard the species as a fictional whole, and to speak of the maintenance of the species as the fictional aim of the processes of reproduction. To go beyond the species with a further fiction of super-individual wholes appears to me inadvisable; I at any rate cannot see what would be gained in our present connection by the fiction of an aim for the whole of life or for the world. Let there be no misunderstanding; there is no intention what-ever here of judging, let alone condemning, those guiding ideas which pedagogics or ethics give to individual persons or to the whole of humanity concerning the meaning and aim of life. In that case the meaning and aim—as I hope to have already made clear—are ideas of value, and hence of entirely different nature from those dealt with here. (For further discussion of the idea of the whole transcending the individual see the seventh and tenth chapters.)

We have already frequently spoken of the human consciousness. It is now time that we should consider this in more detail. Concerning the nature of it, everybody is informed without further explanation; but what the consciousness depends on, and what the meaning of it is, is completely beyond our powers of investigation. We do not know whether in our case it takes an in-dependent part in the processes of our psychical functions. When we make a decision, when we " will " something, it is impossible to decide whether our consciousness produces this act of will out of itself, or whether the act proceeds, in the sense of the mechanistic point of view, as a result of the physiology of the brain, the consciousness being then nothing more than an accompaniment, an " epiphenomenon ".

This brings us to the problem of the freedom of the will. Here again we are dealing with a question fundamentally incapable of decision. For one person, his own freedom of will is directly evident, the other finds it equally obvious that freedom in the common sense—that is, indetermination—is absurd, but that everything must result simply from the physico-chemical processes which form the basis of the physiology of the brain. Both of these views are incapable of proof ; whoever adopts one or the other must be clear about the fact that he is only following the needs of his own individual world attitude, and " laws of logic " which he has created for himself.

Theoretical knowledge that the question of the freedom of the will is insoluble, cannot prevent us from ascribing to the fiction of freedom an important function in social life.

In teaching, criminal law, etc., we cannot do without this fiction ; for it is a very important determining factor in guiding the single individual in a direction desired by human society.

Hence it is impossible for us to decide how human consciousness comes into being ; furthermore, we do not know whether such a thing as freedom of will really exists ; and finally, the question whether an immaterial human psyche also exists or not must remain open. We can only make use of the psyche as a fiction ; we may perhaps be permitted to make use of it as an image.

B

We set up the fiction that behind the life functions of the single organism there stands an immaterial, soul-like agent. Whatever happens in the body is supposed to be under its control, for example, digestion, secretion, breathing, regulation of heat, etc. ; and finally, also the functions of the central nervous system. The latter is again divided into stages of lower and higher centres, the highest layer, in the case of man, being the cortex ; the activity of the latter is connected with the phenomenon of consciousness. We make the further fiction that the psyche-like agent possesses, in the form of this uppermost region of the central nervous system, an instrument, with the help of which it becomes conscious of itself, whereas otherwise it remains hidden and unrecognized by itself. This would make the conscious human psyche the narrow region of the psyche-like agent upon which the spotlight of self-consciousness is able to fall. But do not forget that what I have just put forward is an image, a fiction and nothing more ; in these regions it is impossible to prove anything, all that one can do is to attempt to make that which cannot be directly seen and investigated more or less intelligible by means of comparisons. We are therefore not by any means assuming a contrast between the conscious and the unconscious (or subconscious) in ourselves, as is not uncommonly done. Instead, consciousness shall be for us the continuous prolongation of the unconscious out of darkness into light.

What is now to be said concerning the consciousness of animals ? Here it must be emphasized most decidedly that this again is an insoluble problem. For we do not even know concerning our fellow human beings, anything about the nature of their consciousness and its content. We can only conclude that it is much the same as, or more or less similar, to our own. To take the simplest example, there is no possibility of deciding whether another person experiences the sense of red in exactly the same way as I do. In cases where defective colour vision or even complete colour blindness exists, it is only possible to prove the opposite. The same is true for all other contents of consciousness. In the case of animals, we are quite unable to come to any decision at all; we can only regard it as more or less probable that in their case also something of the kind exists. On the basis of behaviour similar to that of a human being, it may be more or less clear to us that a dog, for example, experiences joy or pain. No proof of this can be given, and the further a species of animals is removed in its organization from our own, the more strange to us is its whole behaviour, and the less are we in a position to feel sympathetically the processes of its consciousness.

The question of animal consciousness must therefore be excluded from animal psychology. Not because it is not interesting, but because it is insoluble. When in these lectures we speak of the purpose of animal behaviour, we therefore can never mean purpose consciously conceived in the animal's psyche, but only a biological end imagined by the observer. In many cases it will follow naturally that this fiction coincides with the conception of purpose in daily life, for example, when any animal makes directly for an object in an unmistakable manner. But the part played by this object in the animal's consciousness, supposing it to be present, cannot be determined. The psyche-like agent which we have imagined as standing behind life processes is, of course, not regarded as " all powerful " and infallible ; it may also " make mistakes ". We have already spoken of processes tending to the destruction of the whole, which occur in disease. Furthermore, in regeneration processes all kinds of malformations occur from time to time ; for example, in the case of newts, the legs may grow too large or too small a number of toes, or limbs may be doubled. Nor does every kind of injury of the organism from outside find suitable regulation ; in many cases therefore, the removal of bodily parts may lead to lifelong injury or early death. Correspondingly, an organism may also make mistakes as regards its loco-motive behaviour towards an external stimulus, par-ticularly when we produce a defect in its sense organs. If for example, we blind an insect on one side, we thus delude it with an apparent darkness on that side, and the result is that when making towards the light it will sometimes not make for it directly, but turn off in arcs and spirals towards its seeing side.

Nevertheless, the animal body always behaves as a whole, even when the functions are not adapted to the situation, as in the case of defective operation in regenera-tion, and in erroneous locomotion. Operation as a whole, and adaptation to the situation, are therefore two different notions. To take an example from human life : in the case of a child that is learning to walk, the body operates as a whole, but not in a manner perfectly adequate to the situation. As the most important result of what has been said in this chapter, I should like to emphasize the following : when we set up the fiction that a psyche-like agent is behind the life function of the individual organism, and creates its character of wholeness, the human psyche will be no more than a part of this which has become conscious of itself. In this way, the contrast between the bodily and psychical functions becomes relative. In the case of animals, we know nothing of a psyche conscious of itself. Nevertheless, the treatment of the subject which we have chosen enables us to deal with all life phenomena in animals : metabolism, growth, regeneration, locomotion, and so on, under a single point of view.

CHAPTER III

Individuality—the ciliated slipper-animalcule (*Paramecium*) as individual.

WE will commence our survey with the concept of individuality. The literal meaning of " individual " is that which is indivisible. In the case of man and the higher animals indivisibility is largely a fact. It may first be said that we experience ourselves subjectively at every moment as an indivisible unity. Certain parts of the body, for example, arms or legs, can be removed from man or higher animals, without his life being directly endangered thereby ; but the part cut off perishes. Such an operation, therefore, does not give us two parts each capable of separate life. And if we were to attempt to cut one of the higher organisms into two parts of approximately equal size, we should be met with complete failure, inasmuch as both halves would then immediately perish. However, by suitable treatment it is possible to maintain alive for a considerable time parts separated from the bodies of the higher and even the highest animals. The isolated heart, for example, of a frog or other vertebrate continues to beat if we supply it with a suitable salt solution in place of blood. Success has also been obtained in removing parts of the bodies of higher vertebrates—for example chicken embryos, and cultivating them further in artificial media. In this way, it is possible to maintain for a long period cultures of

22

connective tissue, muscle-cells, epithelia, gland cells, and so on, and even to cause them to multiply greatly. Nevertheless, the characteristic structure of the organs in question, which would otherwise be built up by these cells, is lost, and the cells themselves may change their nature very greatly. They grow into nothing more than an irregular mass of cells. All the same, we are obliged to conclude that even the highest organism is not indivisible in the strictest sense, since it is possible to grow single parts of its structure in a suitable culture medium ; this method is called " explantation ".

As regards the lower animals, in many cases there can be no question of indivisibility. Many protozoa can be cut up in various ways ; the parts remain alive and regenerate themselves to complete animals ; it is, however, necessary that each such part should contain some nuclear tissue. In the case of an amœba having a single nucleus, only that part continues to live which contains the nucleus ; amœbæ which have many nuclei regenerate from all parts which contain at least one nucleus. In the case of Stentor (one of the ciliates, so called from its trumpet-like form), the nucleus is shaped like a chain of pearls ; if we cut such an animal into several parts, all those regenerate which contain a portion of the nucleus. As regards lower multi-cellular animals, for example a freshwater polyp (Hydra) or many worms, we have already said that they can be cut up into very many parts, and that each part is capable of developing into a complete animal. By natural means also, two or more animals may arise out of one ; the multiplication of protozoa takes place by means of such cell-division. In many classes of multi-cellular animals, we find, along with sexual reproduction, reproduction by budding, in which one animal forms as a bud on another, from which it finally separates itself. If this complete independence is not reached, that is, if the individuals formed as buds remain physically connected with the parents, we have the formation of "colonies", where in extreme cases the single individual actually becomes some special organ of the colony, and the colony itself then takes the rank of an individual. As regards plants, everyone knows that a large number of species are mainly propagated by cuttings.

The opposite process to the division of individuality into two or more parts is the artificial union of two parts derived from different animals to form a single whole. Graftings of this kind have been successful in the case of the multi-nuclear amœba Pelomyxa, and of Hydra, earthworms, and amphibia spores, etc. The part played by grafting in gardening needs no emphasis.

Individuality in biology cannot therefore be defined as indivisibility. Individuality can rather only be regarded as the functioning with reference to a whole of those parts of an organism which are connected together in a normal manner. All functions are to be included, thus metabolism, growth, bodily movement and locomotion, etc. If the normal connection between the various regions of the body is destroyed, the wholeness of the functions is correspondingly vitiated.

So far we have not only considered the reactions of animals as regards movement, but also all other possible phenomena of life, such as metabolism, growth, reproduction, and regeneration. This was done to show that bodily movement and locomotion do not occupy a special position as regards the animal's performance, but that all its life processes may be regarded from a single point of view. But from now on attention will be mainly directed to the particular theme of this book, the science of the behaviour of animals. We will begin with the protozoa, and test by means of several examples whether the fictions we have set up of wholeness and relation to the whole, etc., are applicable to the behaviour of these unicellulare creatures.

We will only deal shortly with the amœba. It is generally visible to the naked eye, and crawls about the bottom under water by stretching out foot-like appendages (pseudopods) in one direction and drawing them in in the other. This means of locomotion only gives the impression of complete irregularity when considered quite superficially. It can only be understood as a function of the whole; for if the motion of the pseudopods were not always concerted, every amœba would very soon tear itself into a number of small parts. The amœba, also, always reacts as a whole whenever it meets on its way a stimulus which causes it to change its direction. A chemical stimulus, one of heat or touch, or sudden illumination, will all serve this purpose. The amœba is therefore not merely a lump of protoplasm, without definite form, but more than that: an individual in the sense of our definition.

We will now treat at greater length another example from the protozoa, the *Paramecium*. This belongs to the class of ciliates, and is completely covered with several thousand fine hairs (cilia), which are able to move rapidly. The animal, which, like the amœba, consists only of a single cell, has a length of about one-hundrèdth of an inch, and is therefore just visible to the naked eye. Its body is approximately cigar-shaped ; we are able to distinguish a back and a belly. In the latter we find the mouth, which is prolonged to form a cavity which receives the particles of nourishment supplied to the cell body. The mouth lies at the end of the mouth-region, which begins on the left side of the front end of the body, and passes diagonally backwards as a flat depression. The presence of this depression leads to the Paramecium bearing a distant resemblance to a slipper, hence the name slipper-animalcule. The mouth region makes the cell body slightly asymmetrical.

The animal's locomotive apparatus is the covering of cilia. The cilia are planted in the surface of the body and each springs from a swelling or root, the "basal granule." Not only in the case of Paramecium, but in the case of other animals, these two structures, the cilium and its basal granule, are described as the cilium element, and when we isolate such an element, it is able to move on its own account for a short time, until it finally perishes. If, on the other hand, we separate the cilium from its root, it immediately comes to rest. There is an important difference between the beat of the single cilium element when isolated and when situated in its normal position on the body. The motion of the isolated cilium is invariable or stereotyped ; the only change that one observes is that it first moves at a furious speed, then gradually tires, and finally comes to rest. As opposed to this stereotyped motion of an isolated element we have the motion of the cilia on an intact Paramecium; sometimes they beat quickly, sometimes more slowly and sometimes they stand still. Obviously something is present which regulates the activity of the individual ciliæ.

When we observe an uninjured Paramecium under the microscope, we can make another important observation regarding its hairy coat; the movements of the single cilia do not happen independently of one another. There is always a connection between them, such that those standing behind one another, in the direction of the stroke, swing in turn one after another (metachronously), whereas those which are alongside one another swing together (synchonously). This process gives much the same impression as we get from a field of corn over which gusts of wind are blowing, and causing the corn to move in waves.

The Paramecium either remains at rest, or moves according to the number of its cilia which beat, and according to the strength with which they do so. We see a picture which continually changes; at one moment the animal is still, and attaches itself by means of a number of its cilia, which are then held rigid, to some object. Only the cilia around the mouth are then in motion, bringing particles of food to the animal; but this process may be helped by a larger or smaller number of the other hairs co-operating. Then most of the cilia, or all of them, may suddenly begin to work very actively, and the animal swims away.

The forward motion of the Paramecium, like that of

the other ciliates, is, in free water, a rotatory. The animal thus moves screw-fashion, that is, in a spiral, the front part describing a larger circle than the other end. The animal turns, as seen from the front, clockwise. Its back is always directed outwards, and its belly towards the axis of its rotation. Let us suppose that an individual which we are observing meets in the course of swimming with some stimulus, for example, some chemical dissolved in the water. The animal then has a number of different possibilities by which it can avoid the irritant. It may carry out a searching movement, stopping for a moment and moving its fore-part in a circle, the whole body thus moving round the surface of an imaginary cone ; after this, the animal may set off in another direction. Or the animal avoids the dissolved substance by going around it in a curve, and returning to its old surroundings. It can carry out its avoiding movement still more quickly by suddenly turning aside, or even completely round. If the stimulus is very strong, the Paramecium may move backwards for a space, rotating as in the case of its forward motion, and in the same direction. It will then change over to swimming forwards in another direction.

These by no means exhaust all the ways in which the paramecium may move. It may also travel forwards without rotation, as it frequently does when moving over a surface. And when it moves in a medium which has been thickened, for example, by quince-mucilage, it no longer turns clockwise, but in the opposite direction. The biological meaning of this change in its rotation is by no means clear.

All these different ways of moving forward are effected by the activity of the cilia. If the animal is moving forwards and rotating clockwise, the cilia work correspondingly in a sideway direction, or that is to say, if we are looking at the animal, they move to the right and backwards; if it is moving forwards without rotating, they all beat together forwards and backwards. If the animal is moving backwards and rotating, the cilia have to move sideways and forwards, and when it is moving forwards in a thick medium and rotating in the opposite direction, the cilia have to move to the left and backwards. We can convince ourselves by observing the animal under the microscope that it moves forward as a whole in a manner corresponding to the way in which the cilia are working. In the more complicated types of motion however, as described above—the searching movement around a cone, the swimming in a curve and the sudden turn from a stimulus—it is impossible to observe accurately how the cilia move.

But whether we are able to observe the direction of beat in detail or not, one thing is certain : in all cases the whole of the cilia—and this means, as I have said, many thousands of single hairs—move in strict co-ordination ; single cilia never work independently of the others, as they do when separated from the body. But how is this co-ordination brought about ? In higher animals and man we have, in the central nervous system, a clearly distinguishable centre which takes care of the activity of the locomotive organs, for example the legs. A special centre of this kind is wanting in the bodies of protozoa, and nevertheless we observe the strictly co-ordinated working of the many thousand locomotive elements, the cilia.

We can come to no other conclusion than that, in the case of the protozoa, the whole cell acts as its own central organ for control of locomotion ; according to this view, it depends upon the whole condition of the Paramecium cell at any time, which of the cilia beat, and which remain at rest. Single cilia, or any particular collection of them, never answer independently to any stimulus from outside. Such a stimulus is first transmitted to the whole cell, and this decides whether, and how, and by what cilia, the stimulus is to be met. The single cilium is only able on its own account to produce a purely stereotyped beat ; according to the situation, the whole condition of the cell protoplasm checks, releases, or otherwise regulates the motion of the single hairs, and thus turns their individual activities into a total activity regulated as a whole.

When natural cell division commences, a constriction is formed in the middle of the body of the Paramecium, which at first does not prevent the activity of the hairs from being in unison. But as the circular depression becomes deeper and deeper, a moment comes when the individuality originally existing begins to separate into two. This moment is apparent to the observer by the fact that differences appear in the activity of the cilia of the two animals—the fore and hind parts. Finally, the two twins are only connected by a fine thread of proto- plasm ; but the co-ordination in beat between the fore part and the hind part is then already at an end ; one may be at rest, while the other sets its cilia working, the former being dragged forward for a little by the latter, until it itself begins to swim actively. Or both may have their cilia working actively, and pull one another to and fro, until finally the connecting thread breaks and we have two entirely independent individuals.

Division of this kind can be imitated artificially. By means of a fine thread of glass we can cut a Paramecium into two halves, the fore part and the hind part; both parts then swim away in different directions. All relation between them has ceased to exist; each half-animal exhibits, as regards the activity of its cilia, unity of action. In forward motion, therefore, both halves rotate clockwise; after a stimulus, for example, by touch, they move, rotating in the same sense, backwards a short distance. If we thicken the medium by means of gum, both the fore-animal and the hind-animal rotate counter-clockwise. In all these cases we see that, as in the case of an intact individual, the whole coating of hairs works in unison in corresponding direction. The isolated half-animals are also able to come to rest for a time, whereupon the cilia are stationary. The fact that the two half-animals usually perish in a short time, about one half to one hour, has no importance in this connection. This fact depends mainly upon the size of the wound. But in any case, and at the very best, only one half would be capable of survival, since only one half can be in possession of the nucleus. It is, by the way, of importance that the motion of the cilia in the two halves takes place without reference to the presence or absence of nuclear substance; the nucleus is therefore not responsible for the production of ciliary motion and its various modifications.

The experiment of artificially dividing the Paramecium into two individuals can be varied by not completely cutting the animal in half, but merely compressing it strongly in the middle of its body by means of the glass thread. If by this means we succeed in abolishing the granular structure of the protoplasm at this point, the front and hind halves each operate on their own account, and give separate impulses to the cilia attached to them. Harmony then only exists as a secondary matter; when, for example, one half drives the whole body forward by active motion of the cilia, the other half usually takes up the same activity; but this is in no way the result of the conduction of an impulse along the protoplasm, but obviously is caused by a purely mechanical stimulus, due to the half in question being pulled passively through the water. And at any moment the co-operation may come to an end by one of the halves changing the character of its ciliary motion.

If we observe an animal thus crushed in the middle for a somewhat longer time, we see that the structure of the protoplasm reappears in about half an hour at the point of injury. This depends upon the fact that the protoplasm flows together in front and back halves, and in the same degree as this takes place co-ordination between the fore part and the hind part is renewed, so that at the end of the process we have again to deal with an individual which acts with complete unity. Our interference therefore divided the individuality of the Paramecium into two parts; but after a short time these two were again united and became one.

What has been said above concerning the Paramecium

evidently holds in principle for all ciliates, and indeed for all protozoa. According to their bodily organization, their modes of reaction and behaviour of course differ; but we are always dealing with living creatures which, exactly like the higher animals, take rank as organisms possessed of an individuality. While, therefore, an unbridgeable gap separates living from non-living nature, the differences between various living creatures appear to be of a more gradual description.

We may deal shortly with some other ciliates. Stentor, which we have already mentioned, is more complicated in structure than Paramecium. It possesses two kinds of cilia; one a general coat of hairs covering the body uniformly, and the second a spiral of cilia which surrounds the mouth at the fore part of the body. This spiral consists of little bundles of cilia arranged one behind the other, and these, when the animal takes hold anywhere with its hinder part, waft particles of nourishment to its mouth. When the animal lets go, they assist the other cilia to produce locomotion. A peculiarity of Stentor is the possession of muscular fibres running lengthwise along the body, and enabling the animal to contract with lightning rapidity, when stimulated. The statement made by earlier writers, that Stentor also possesses nerve threads, has not been confirmed.

Stentor swims with a clockwise rotation; if it meets an obstacle, it is, like Paramecium, able to avoid this in many different ways. It may continue to rotate in the same sense, but move backwards for a space, and then proceed to swim forward again in another direction; or it may avoid the obstacle in a more direct manner by

c

describing a curve with its fore part; a curve of this kind may carry the animal completely round to the opposite direction.

Spirostomum is a relative of Stentor. This has a body which is over two millimetres long, and about one-fifth of a millimetre broad, and is thus thread or worm-like. Its possession of muscular fibres renders it highly capable of contraction; when it comes up against any kind of resistance, the animal can move its fore part tentatively to and fro, until it finds a way out. In other cases Spirostomum, when it strikes upon an object, can move the fore part of its body exactly like a worm, and glide past the obstacle. In another infusorium of this class (*Loxophyllum*) we may have, according to the situation in which the animal finds itself, both investigatory motion of the fore point of the body, and wavelike movement of the whole, as well as the most various twists and turns.

We may say, to sum up: even the protozoa, which have been described as the " lowest " animals, since their body consists " only of a single cell ", do not react in an automatic and stereotyped way to the peculiarities of the external medium, but rather—of course in accordance with their organization—as whole individuals, and in a manner highly variable and suited to the situation. In their case, a single cell executes all that in other animals, and man, can only be done by millions and milliards of cells acting together. Regarded " from the protozoan point of view " we can also say that for this reason these single-celled creatures must be regarded as the " highest " organisms. A central organ differentiated in structure, and capable of maintaining unity of behaviour, is missing in the case of the protozoan cell; and hence we are obliged to regard the cell body as a whole as its own centre, which then sends suitable impulses, according to the nature of the situation, to the various cell organs.

CHAPTER IV

More concerning the individuality of animals possessing numerous like organs of locomotion.—The free-swimming Turbellaria and Starfish.

In the last chapter we dealt with the unicellular animals, the protozoa. We chose as our main example Paramecium, and saw that it possesses, in the form of its cilia, many thousands of exactly similar locomotive organs, each of which, when separated from connection with the body, carries out independent motion of a completely stereotyped kind. On the other hand, as long as it is connected in a normal manner with the living cell, it always obeys the unitary impulses proceeding therefrom. In the case also of multicellular animals, the metazoa, we frequently meet with the possession of cilia, which cover, to a greater or lesser extent, the surface or the internal cavities of the body. In smaller forms of metazoa, which live in water, this ciliary coat covering the body frequently serves for locomotion, and we will now see whether, in these cases as well, it is subjected to unitary central impulses.

Speaking quite generally, the bodies of metazoa exhibit a division of labour among the cells, which finds its expression in a variety of structure. The nerve cells act as the central organ ; only in the case of the sponges are they absent. In the case of freshwater polyps (*Hydra*) and their related forms, they are distributed fairly uniformly in the body, being connected with one another by nerve threads; they thus form a diffuse central nervous system. But in the animal kingdom, a compact central nervous system is commonest, and we find at least the vast majority of the nerve cells concentrated in definite regions of the body; in vertebrates, for example, in the form of the brain and spinal cord. We then only find a small number of nerve cells in other parts of the body, for example, in the heart or intestines. These give the organs in question a certain independence in their activity; but these peripherally situated nerve cells are by no means completely independent as regards transmission of impulses, but are connected by nerves with the rest of the central nervous system, and are always under the control of the latter.

Also in the case of the metazoa, the cilium element is formed of the single hair and its root. The cilia are collected in considerable numbers on the surface of the so-called ciliary cells, and these are then united to form larger aggregates, the ciliary epithelia, which may be of quite different sizes, from case to case. As long as no disturbance occurs from outside, the activity of the cilia, both those on an individual cell, and upon the whole ciliary epithelium, is perfectly co-ordinated. That is to say, they beat in a single direction, those alongside one another beating, as in the case of the infusoria, together (synchronously), while those behind one another beat in succession (metachronously), so that uniform waves of motion pass over the ciliary epithelium.

Epithelia of this kind may, according to the nature of the animal, have various biological " duties " (the concept

" duty " being, of course, meant in the fictional sense). We are able to distinguish two kinds of ciliary epithelia according to their function ; one kind works invariably, and always, in one and the same direction, and is free from the influence of the central nervous system. In this class we have, for example, the epithelia which cover the inner surface and gills of shell-fish ; they transport particles of nourishment, which were embedded in the mud, towards the mouth. In the case of snails, which move along a path of slime which they produce themselves, the cilia distributed upon the lower surface of the animal take care that the secretion of slime is uniformly distributed. In man, also, we find ciliary epithelia, for example, in the air passages to the lungs ; the motion of the cilia is directed towards the nostrils, and its purpose is to transport mucus, and the small foreign bodies contained in it, outwards from the body. Ciliary epithelium of this kind, in which the beat of the cilia takes place unchanged in one and the same direction, and is independent of the influence of the central nervous system, may be described as the irregulatory type.

As opposed to this, we have the regulatory type, in which the motion is subjected to a central influence. In this class belong the infusoria, for we saw that in their case the activity of the cilia is regulated by the whole cell. Both regulatory and irregulatory epithelia may actually occur in one and the same species of metazoa, for example, in many water snails. Where we have regulatory cilia they usually serve for locomotion, and allow the animals to swim about freely in water.

We may take as our illustration the native turbellarians,

which live in water, and the smaller and almost microscopic species of which possess regulatory, and the large species irregulatory cilia. The first-mentioned forms are rod-like, the latter are flattened and rather leaf-like. The central nervous system of turbellarians consists of a pair of ganglia situated at the fore-part, and nerve-cords running backwards; the possession of numerous muscles gives the body of the animal great power of motion. In the case of animals covered with irregulatory cilia, the beat is always directed backward; the species in question creep in the manner of snails along the bottom of the water in a path of slime which they secrete, locomotion not being effected by the cilia situated on their lower surface, but by very fine muscular motions. The cilia situated on the rest of the body surface produce a continual current of water past the animal, which serves on the one hand for breathing, and on the other hand for the discovery of prey. The beat of the cilia always remains the same, whether the individual is at rest, moving straight forwards, or moving in a curve, etc.

Matters are quite otherwise in the case of free-swimming turbellarians, which possess regulatory cilia. Here the covering of hairs serves for locomotion, and works exactly in the manner with which we are already familiar from the infusoria, namely, in unison, and in the most variable modes of response to the momentary situation. And not only is there the strictest agreement between the activity of the various cilia, but also between ciliary motion and muscular contraction. It is quite evident that both systems of organs receive at the same moment co-ordinated impulses, which in this case, where a central nervous system exists, must obviously be regarded as proceeding from it.

By means of a narcotic we are able, both in the case of free-swimming and of creeping turbellarians, to put the central nervous system out of action for a certain time. In every case muscular motion then ceases, and the bodies of the individuals remain stiff and motionless as long as insensibility continues. Ciliary motion, on the other hand, does not cease. Worms which normally creep lose, under a narcotic, contact with the bottom, and are then driven through the water by the backward, stereotyped beat of their ciliary covering, until they strike against some object and are thus held up; but their cilia continue to work uninterruptedly. Recovery from the narcotic is signalized by single muscular contractions; these gradually become more frequent, and the animal finally makes an active endeavour to regain contact with the bottom; and then, completely awake, proceeds to creep about in the usual manner.

In one of the free-swimming turbellarians, a narcotic leads to the central nervous system losing control both over the muscles and over the cilia. As a result of the stiffening of the muscle the body becomes like a piece of wood, the variability of the ciliary motion ceases, and gives place to a completely stereotyped beat. In other words, during narcosis the impulses cease, which normally change the ciliary motion from moment to moment, and suit it to the immediate situation; the ciliary elements become autonomous, but are only able to carry out on their own account a stereotyped beat—a fact already known to us from the isolated ciliary elements of Paramecium. In these narcotized worms, the cilia beat sideways and backwards; as a result, the body moves forwards with a clockwise rotation. Since the animal is not able to avoid obstacles, it arrives sooner or later in a corner and remains there until it gradually recovers from the narcotic. Its reawakening is heralded by muscular contractions, which mainly lead to the animal freeing itself, on meeting an obstacle, by suitable twists of its body. After a short time, modification of the beat of the cilia begins, together with stronger muscular contractions, and finally, the individual returns to its normal condition.

We have therefore succeeded in eliminating by narcosis in the case of the freely swimming turbellarians, the influence of central nervous system, which is well defined anatomically. But is it therefore permissible for us to say that we have been able to turn the turbellarian during narcosis into an infusorian-like creature? It is easy to see that such a view would be completely wrong; for, though it is true that the infusorian is devoid of a separate central organ, it possesses such an organ to all intents and purposes, inasmuch as the whole of its protoplasm forms such a centre, from which impulses proceed to the cilia according to the momentary situation. The uninjured infusorian is therefore a complete organism with all necessary qualities and powers; the narcotized worm, on the other hand, is incomplete in one important respect, namely the power of its central nervous system to function.

In the case of the infusoria and free-swimming turbellaria therefore, the locomotive apparatus consists of a large

number of similar parts, the cilia. In this connection
we may discuss another group of animals, whose motor
system differs very widely from the forms we have been
considering; but nevertheless possesses a feature in
common, namely, that here also a large number of
similarly constructed elements, working together in a
co-ordinated manner, bring about steady motion of the
whole animal. I am referring to the echinoderms, of
which at least the sea-urchin and the starfish will be
known to you. These animals, in contrast to the majority
of other animals, are not bilaterally symmetrical, but
constructed on a starlike plan. It is possible to divide
their bodies by means of several—most frequently five—
imaginary planes, each of which separates into halves
which are mirror-images of one another. The most
obvious example of this is afforded by the five-ray symmetry of the starfish, the body of which is prolonged
into five arms. A chalky skeleton gives its body a certain
rigidity; but this skeleton is divided into numerous
parts which are capable of relative motion, so that the
animal is able to use its muscles to bend and twist in
all sorts of ways. The mouth is situated centrally on
the lower side; and from it a furrow extends along
each arm. The central nervous system and the locomotor
system are likewise situated on the lower side of the body.
The former, in the case of the starfish, is not situated
inside the body, as in the case of most other animals,
but is freely exposed on the underside. It consists of
a ring of nerves which surrounds the mouth, and five
radial nerves belonging to each of the five arms. In the
region of the mouth, and in the furrows running along

the rays, are many hundreds of minute feet, each of which carries a sucker at its outer end. These feet are characterized by great mobility, and are able to stretch out and withdraw. They are hollow, and filled with a liquid; each foot possesses a cavity which extends into the body, and which, when contraction occurs, takes up the excess of liquid. All the feet of one arm are connected by a longitudinal tube, the radial water vessel, which, alongside the radial nerve, runs along the furrow of the arm; and the five radial vessels are connected among themselves by means of a circular canal which runs along the mouth. Functioning of the feet occurs as the result of impulses sent out by the central nervous system; as the starfish creeps, it plants its feet in one and the same direction against the bottom, stretches them, and thus pushes its body in the opposite direction. The feet then release themselves from the bottom, swing back, and proceed to take another step in the manner described. Accordingly as the feet work alternately or in unison, the motion is continuous or in jerks. The animal is able to creep in any direction with reference to its body, the single arms then being stretched or curved in the most various ways.

We must not underestimate the achievement of the animal in being able to co-ordinate all its feet and cause them to operate in one and the same direction. Let us first consider those feet which belong to one and the same arm. Let us imagine these first stretched straight out, the radial nerves lying in the long axis. All the feet, in performing their to-and-fro movement, are set at the same angle to the nerve, as seen from above. But as soon as an arm is bent during locomotion, the individual feet may form, seen from above, the most various angles with the respective nerve. The matter becomes still more complicated when we consider feet belonging to different arms; for these have to take up with respect to the long axis of their arms entirely different angles, if they are to press against the ground in such a way as to act always in the same direction.

The common feature, as I have said, of starfish, free-swimming turbellarians, and Paramecium, is that their locomotor apparatus consists of a large number of similar individual elements, the feet or cilia as the case may be, and that these, by working in strict co-ordination, produce a unitary movement of the entire body. These animals also, therefore, supply us with examples of our two fictional rules: " The end determines the means ", and " The whole determines the parts ". For " whole ", and " end ", are in both cases the total locomotion in a definite direction; and to these are subordinated the " means ", or the " parts ", that is to say the motion of the individual feet or cilia as the case may be, to meet the momentary situation.

If we turn a starfish on its back it bends the points of its rays round until the feet upon them are able to touch the bottom. The feet of one arm then begins to contract and to pull over the body, whereby more and more feet belonging to this arm are able to take firm hold of the bottom; the arms on the other side assist the process by pressing against the bottom and thus levering the body over. In this manner, the starfish is able to regain its normal position in a very short space of time.

Some have wished to discern opposition in the functioning of the five arms in the fact that the starfish at first generally bends all its arms, and so brings the feet at their points in contact with the ground. The five single arms were thus regarded as five individuals, and each was supposed to begin to operate in a particular direction. The final overturn was then supposed to come about by a compromise between the five forces opposing one another. In an extreme form this was formulated as follows : the " I " of the starfish is made up of a " We ", of the single " I's " of the five arms ; this was described as the " We in the I ". Of course, the reference to an " I " was purely metaphorical ; the starfish was not supposed to possess a conscious ego. Nevertheless, this view is certainly to be rejected. For as far as one can see, the five arms do not behave like five draught animals, harnessed to a cart and striving to move it in five different directions, the decision as to the direction of motion of the cart being given by the relative strength of the animals. We do not assume a functional opposition between the right- and the left-hand side of the body in the case of an organism which is bilaterally symmetrical, and we have no more right to assume such an opposition between the similarly constructed parts of a five-rayed animal. If we lay a bilaterally symmetrical organism, for instance, an insect, a crab, or a frog, upon its back, it usually performs, during the first moments, grasping or searching movements with all its extremities, until they have found a hold upon the ground or upon some solid object ; whereupon the animal immediately turns over with a single unitary movement. Accordingly, we must regard the bending of the starfish's rays as exploratory movements, which enable it to discover a hold ; as soon as it has found this, co-ordinated impulses proceed to all necessary parts of the body : the muscles, which move the arms, and the feet. Thus, its regaining a normal position appears from beginning to end as a completely unitary act.

If we cut a starfish into two or more parts, we divide its individuality in the corresponding manner. Each single isolated arm is capable of continued existence ; it crawls about and finally regenerates four new arms, and in the end becomes a complete starfish. If we divide the ring of nerves surrounding the mouth at two points, without otherwise injuring the animal, we obtain two half-animals which are completely independent as regards their central nervous system ; within themselves these two parts act in perfect co-ordination, but as regards one another they exhibit no further functional relationship, in spite of the fact that they are still mechanically connected. Locomotion, overturn, and so on, now only result in a compromise between two forces acting independently of one another. This contrast between animals in which the central nervous system has been divided into two, and intact starfish, exhibits to us, in the clearest possible manner, the fact that all the movements of the latter always take place in a unitary manner.

By way of conclusion we may consider the sea-urchin. Its body is spherical ; but we are able clearly to distinguish in it five-rayed symmetry. The function of its feet is another than in the case of the starfish, for they do not push the animal forward by stretching, but pull it forward by contraction. But the same is true in principle for the sea-urchin as for the starfish; if the animal is on the move, its feet swing to-and-fro in one and the same direction in space; but with respect to the particular fifth section of the body to which they belong, this direction is in each case a different one, and when the animal changes the direction of its march, the mode of motion of its feet must change in a corresponding manner. The sea-urchin, as compared with the starfish, possesses still another means of locomotion: walking on its spines, and this usually occurs under strong stimulus, and enables the animal to move faster than when using its feet.

The spines of the sea-urchin are longer than those of the starfish, and extremely mobile; when used for locomotion they are swung to and fro, and as regards the relationship of this movement to the divisions of the body upon which the spines are situated, we may say the same as we have said in reference to the motion of the feet.

CHAPTER V

The individuality of jointed animals, annelids, and arthropods.—
The supposed antagonism between the right and left side of
the body.—Theories of tropism, and the theory of tropotaxis.

ACCORDING to the definition we have given, individuality
is not a matter of the indivisibility of the organism, but
of the unitary operation, in undisturbed connection, of
all the parts. We have hitherto dealt in greater detail
with the slipper animalcule (Paramecium), the free-
swimming turbellaria, and the starfish. These various
animal forms, in themselves entirely different, have this
in common, that their locomotion is effected by a large
number of similar single organs : in the case of Paramecium and turbellaria, these were the cilia, and in the
case of the starfish the suckers. These examples made
it particularly evident that the process of locomotion
can never be understood from the individual motions
alone, but only as a unitary function of the whole. We
will now consider animals the bodies of which are built
up out of a number of parts which are completely or
closely similar in construction, and arranged one behind
the other ; such animals are the annelids. They are
known to everyone by at least one species, the earthworm
(*Lumbricus*).

As the name indicates, the bodies of the annelids are
made up of a number of separate rings or segments,
the majority of which are identical in form both externally

48

and internally ; the organs, therefore, both on the exterior
and interior of each segment, are the same in all. At
the front end we find a more or less elaborately constructed
head, which in the case of many species living in water,
may possess feelers, eyes, and other organs. In this
connection we are particularly interested in the nature
of the muscular and central nervous system. The former
consists in both annular and longitudinal muscles, which
lie in the wall of the body. The annular muscles diminish
by their contraction the diameter of the segment to which
they belong, and cause it to increase in length. The
longitudinal muscles operate as antagonists of the annular
muscles, that is to say, their contraction shortens the
segment, and increases its diameter. The central nervous
system of the annelids is built on the plan of a rope
ladder ; a system of this kind occurs, by the way, not
only in this type, but also in the arthropods, which also
possess segmental bodies ; the insects and crayfish
belonging to this class.

It is characteristic of this type of nervous system,
that each segment of the body possesses on the ventral
side a pair of ganglia ; and these contain the nerve cells.
The two ganglia are connected together by a nerve cord ;
and connection also exists between the ganglia of neighbouring segments. It is thus that we get the plan of
a rope ladder. In the head we get two special pairs of
ganglia, the supra and infra-œsophageal. The first lies,
in accordance with its name, above, and the second
below the beginning of the gut ; the connection between
the upper and lower ganglia is made by the œsophageal
connection to right and left of the intestine. The upper

D

pair of ganglia is called, in the case of the annelids and arthropods, the brain, since it is the seat of the highest nerve centres. Secondarily, the two ganglia in each segment of the body may combine to form a single structure, so that the rope ladder becomes a cord extending along below the intestine, with a swelling at each segment brought about by the union of the two ganglia. At the fore end this cord divides into the two connections which proceed to the brain. In the case of earthworms, each pair of ganglia controls that segment to which it belongs. We will first consider an annelid living in the sea, *Nereis*. This worm grows to several centimetres in length, and since it occurs along all our coasts it can easily be sent alive from one of the marine research stations. Its body is constructed of almost a hundred similarly formed segments ; the front end is formed by the head. The section of an individual segment is not circular, but elongated, since it bears to right and left a movable projection which carries a number of bristles. These stump-like projections (parapodia or parapods) are the organs of locomotion.

Nereis lives in the find mud, and moves forward by creeping in it ; it is also able to leave the bottom and swim for a space, though not very skilfully. Its slowest type of crawl consists in the body remaining stretched straight out, and in the passage of waves of motion over the parapods on the right and left side. The animal thus moves forward over the bottom. In this type of metachronous motion, neighbouring parapods are therefore never in like phase of activity, the more forward parapod is always a little in advance, in its motion, of the one behind it. It is also important that the parapods to left and right of the same segment are as a rule functioning in opposite phases. The metachronous waves passing along the right and left of the animal's body remind us of the moment of the cilia of Paramecium and of other such organisms, in which, as we have seen, elements lying behind one another are similarly different in phase.

When an animal at rest begins to creep slowly forwards, the wave motions of the parapods may begin at any part of its body, and not necessarily at the fore part; the waves do not always proceed as far as the hinder part, but may end at any part of the body. By an action of this kind, the animal is able to move very slowly over the bottom. While the co-ordinated function of the cilia of Paramecium is governed by the whole cell, and in a free-swimming turbellarian by the central nervous system, in the case of Nereis the metachronous movement of the parapods depends upon the central nervous system. If the worm, when crawling, meets a resistance of any kind, it may move backwards for a space; this is brought about by a reversal of the motion of the parapod; but in this case also, the parapod situated nearer the head is in advance in its motion as regards that of a parapod situated nearer the tail.

The forward creep of Nereis is more rapid when the animal makes snake-like movements in conjunction with the functioning of its parapods. When this happens, the parapods on its convex side are always in the phase of backward movement and those on the concave side perform their forward motion. The snake-like motion

along the bottom may pass over into swimming, whereupon the movements, which are still performed in the
horizontal plane, become livelier and greater in extent.
When a resting animal is stimulated by being touched
suddenly, it makes use, as a reaction of its body as a
whole, of the contractile reflex, by means of which it
contracts with lightning rapidity. If we divide the
central nervous system of a Nereis at any point, which
is an easy matter, we divide the worm thus into a " fore-
animal " and a " hind-animal ", which are then completely
independent as regards central nervous reaction, and are
only connected in a purely mechanical manner. We
have divided the individuality of the worm into two
parts. It then happens that the fore-animal and the
hind-animal may be acting in entirely different ways,
without any connection with one another. For example,
the former may creep along the bottom, while the latter
is inactive, and hence is passively towed behind the other.
Or the hind-animal may be in motion, and the fore-animal
at rest, a state of affairs which, however, is more seldom
realized, since the fore-animal possesses the highest
centres localized in the brain, and hence is characterized
by greater liveliness. The mode of motion of one half
of the animal may be secondarily transmitted to the
other half ; for example, the resting hind-animal may be
carried forward passively for a space, which process
then results in stimuli of various kinds, and finally lead
the hind-animal also to make locomotive motions. Thus
we may have, for a time, more or less unitary creeping
or swimming, until one or other of the half-animals
returns to a state of rest. This state of inactivity then

either extends to the other half as well—probably on
account of the powerful mechanical resistance given by
the drag of the other half; or, on the other hand, the
inactivity of the resting half lasts only for a short time,
since the persistent activity of the other half causes it
to begin to move again.

Exactly corresponding results are obtained when we
divide the individuality of the worm into three parts,
by cutting the central nervous system at two points.
We may take for further experiments the earthworm
(*Lumbricus*). This is fundamentally similar in construction
to the Nereis. Its body consists of well over one hundred
segments ; it is, however, devoid of a well-developed head
and the extensions to the segments known as parapods.
Hence its section is approximately circular. When
creeping over the ground, it takes hold by means of fine
bristles, which are situated, regularly arranged, on the
lower side of each segment. One can observe the presence
of these bristles by laying an earthworm on its back
and stroking its belly from front to back with the finger.
The creeping motion of the earthworm begins with an
extension and stretching of the forward end. The resulting
contraction of the body passes as a wave backwards
along it and is followed by a thickening and shortening
of the segments ; in this way the forward creeping earthworm exhibits several waves of thinning and thickening
directly behind one another, which pass in the form of
peristaltic movements along the body. This peristalsis
is caused by the antagonism between the annular and
longitudinal muscles ; the first effect contraction and
stretching of the segments, the latter thickening and

shortening. In this process, the parts which are stretched move forward a space each time ; they then grip the ground by means of the bristles, and the shortening of the segments then results in forward motion. If an earthworm is stimulated at its fore-end, it either turns aside one way or the other, or it creeps backwards for a space, the sense of the peristalsis being reversed. In this case, the waves of thinning and thickening arise at the hind-end and travel from this forwards over the body, with the result that the animal moves tail forwards. If the earthworm is touched suddenly, it possesses, like Nereis, a contractile reflex as a reaction of the whole body, which draws together with great suddenness.

. By means of a cut through the nerve thread, we can divide the earthworm into a fore and hind animal. Here again we obtain two half-animals entirely independent of one another as regards central nervous reaction. Accordingly, co-ordination of movement between the fore- and hind-ends disappears. For example, a sudden contact causes contraction of only one half and not of the other. Only in one case do we observe, even after severance of the cord, co-ordination between fore- and hind-animals. If the fore-animal commences to move, peristalsis begins at its front end. But when this reaches the point of injury, we are surprised to find that it does not cease there, but passes over into the hind-animal ; the result is that the two half-animals, whose central nervous systems are separated from one another, nevertheless creep forward with uniform rhythm. (Friedländer was the first who made this experiment and some of those subsequently described.) By way of explanation we must assume that peristalsis is not set going by central nervous impulses alone, but that a further process taking place in a reflex manner in each segment is also concerned ; passive extension of the longitudinal muscles of a segment causes active contraction of the corresponding annular muscles ; and this process again brings about active contraction of the longitudinal muscles. A further experiment confirms the fact that this transference of peristalsis from the fore-animal to the hind-animal, after the performance of severance, is a purely mechanical matter. We divide an earthworm into two parts and join the fore- and hind-animal by means of a thread, which may be of any length. The two half-animals then move in complete independence of one another as long as the thread is not tightly stretched. But as soon as this happens, that is to say as soon as the fore-animal drags the hind-animal along for quite a short distance, connection being made by the tightly stretched thread, the hind-animal begins a peristaltic movement, and the two halves creep along with a unitary rhythm. The experimenter is able himself to assume the rôle of the fore-animal ; he may take hold of the thread and exert a tension on the hind-animal. As soon as this is done the latter commences peristaltic motion, beginning from the fore-part, and this continues as long as the thread is pulled. A further variation of this experiment is to connect two intact earthworms by means of a thread, tying the hind-end of one to the fore-end of the other. Invariably, as soon as the thread is stretched and the fore-animal begins to drag the other, co-ordinated loco-motion is set up.

We must not think, however, that experiments of this kind give us a " mechanical explanation " of the creeping of an earthworm. I have already remarked that the mechanical element is only one of two components entering into the locomotion of this worm. It is obvious that the mechanical pull is less important than the central nervous impulses, which first of all set the motion going, and then likewise take care of the further continuation of peristalsis. The fact that the characteristic motion of creeping is also regulated by the central nervous system may be shown in the following manner. We secure an earthworm to a suitable base and remove the whole of the tissue in the middle of the body with the exception of the nerve cord. In this experimental arrangement the worm is unable to move away from its position, but nothing prevents it carrying out peristaltic movements. We now see that the peristalsis which takes place in the fore-end of the animal passes over into the hind-half, although no mechanical pull is exercised on the latter, since the animal is fixed and unable to move. This proves that the central nervous system is also able to maintain peristalsis ; the mechanical pull, the significance of which we have just discussed, is by no means solely decisive, but merely has the task of supporting the central nervous system in its total function by exciting reflexes in the segments. It should be specially emphasized that in the case of the earthworm with its central nervous system severed, a co-ordination between the two halves can only be set up in a purely mechanical way as regards this one activity, namely creeping ; every other kind of co-ordination is entirely abolished after severance.

Hence even animals the bodies of which are built up of a multiplicity of similarly constructed segments, can never be regarded in reference to their behaviour merely as the sum of the parts, but only as wholes. We will now consider the further question whether, in the case of bilaterally symmetrical animals, any activities can be explained additively from the single function of the right and left side of the body; or whether in this case also such an explanation always fails, thus compelling us to regard their behaviour from the point of view of the whole.

Loeb formed the following conception of the manner in which a bilaterally constructed animal attains or avoids a source of stimulus. Suppose, for example, an animal having a right and left eye, such as a worm, crab or insect, is near a lamp, and is striving to reach it. As long as the animal is not symmetrically situated with reference to the stimulus, that is to say, as long as the lamp is not exactly on the prolongation of the axis of its body, one eye is more strongly illuminated than the other. Loeb now assumes that the sense organs of one side, including the eye, are mainly connected through the central nervous system with the muscular organization of the opposite side of the body, so that the optical stimulation of one eye results in the opposite side of the body being chiefly stimulated. Hence, in the case in question, the system of muscles connected with the more intensively illuminated eye would work more powerfully, until the animal came into a symmetrical position with reference to the light. Hence, according to Loeb's theory of *tropism* (as it is called), the behaviour of a bilateral animal is to be explained mainly as resulting from the addition of the functioning of the two sides separately. The locomotion of the animal would thus be effected in much the same way as that of a boat rowed by two oarsmen, one on one side and the other on the other. If the two work with equal power, the boat moves straight forward ; if one rows more strongly, the boat will move in a curve in the opposite direction. Let us consider in detail whether, and how far, the behaviour of animals ever corresponds to the theory of tropism. Let us first take the example in which the animal moves towards a source of stimulus. This is called positive phototaxis. As we have stated, the theory of tropism has it that the legs on the side away from the light work more strongly, until the animal has described a curve and brought itself into a symmetrical position with respect to the light ; from this point the muscles of the right and left leg are equally stimulated, and the animal moves in a straight line towards the light. But if we observe an insect which, to begin with, is unsymmetrically situated with respect to the light, we see that the symmetrical orientation is by no means produced solely by stronger action of the limbs on the side away from the light, causing the animal to be driven in the opposite direction. On the contrary, its turning towards the light has the form of a completely unitary act, in which the legs of the two sides of the body work in co-ordination with one another. It is as if in the boat which we have referred to, we had one man working both oars. If he wishes to cause the boat to turn, he is not limited to causing one oar to work more strongly than the other, but may also proceed to row backwards with one oar and forwards with the other, until the boat points in the desired direction. The insect behaves in precisely the same manner ; it does not only walk in a curve until it sees the light source equally with both eyes, but may at the very beginning jump round with a single movement and take up its final position.

We may now take the case of insects which avoid the light ; their behaviour is called negative phototaxis. Such an animal, also, must as a rule make a turn, but not this time in the direction of the more strongly illuminated eye, but towards the less illuminated. The production of this movement obviously cannot be explained in the same way as the turn in positive phototaxis. On the contrary, Loeb is compelled to assume that, in the case of negative phototaxis, those legs on the opposite side to the more strongly illuminated eye receive less energy than those on the other side.

In order to save his principle that the orientation of bilaterally symmetrical animals comes about by separate working of the two halves of the body, Loeb is driven to this very artificial point of view.

As a further example, we may take a flat-worm, one of the creeping turbellarians already known to us. These animals possess eyes at their fore-end ; let us take a case in which there is one eye on each side. Turbellarians usually avoid light. If we bring such a worm near a light, it turns away from it. This turning motion results, according to the theory of tropism, from one eye receiving more light than the other ; this sends a stronger impulse to the muscles on the opposite side, with the result that they are more strongly contracted, and so bend the animal's body. But when, as may happen, some worm or other strives to reach the light, that is, when we have positive phototaxis, the tropism theory compels us to assume that the half of the body opposite to the illuminated eye receives a less quantity of energy.

In North America, the theory of tropism still possesses a number of adherents; in Germany, various authors (Kühn, O. Koehler, Herter and others) have developed it further into a theory of *tropotaxis*, which, it is true, is an improvement in refinement of its predecessor, but nevertheless is subject to the same fundamental error, namely, that according to it an animal does not react to a source of stimulus in a unitary manner, but additively by the parallel, or even opposed, operation of the right and left side of its body.

Obviously the main reason why the theories of tropism and tropotaxis still find some adherents is that when experiments are done in two dimensions, and the results are represented on paper, the interpretations appear so attractively simple. But if we work in three dimensions, the theories of tropism and tropotaxis inevitably fail. Let us place in a dark room a winged insect upon a table, having placed over the latter a lighted lamp. The insect rises in the air and makes straight for the lamp. How is this possible according to the two theories? For they are only able to explain the guidance of a bilateral organism by the parallel operation of the right and left side of the body in one plane, for example, that of the table; but since the insect is able to leave this plane, and reach a goal, by a diagonal path, is a fact which is entirely overlooked by the two theories. The same is true for water animals, which do not always swim parallel to the earth's surface towards the light, but may, under suitable experimental conditions, also reach it by a movement up or down. These theories are quite unable to deal with all such cases which take place in three-dimensional space, since there is no such thing as a second plane at right angles to the medial plane of the animal's body, and dividing the latter horizontally in two similar halves. For the reasons we have given, the theories of tropism and tropotaxis must be rejected ; above all, they contradict fundamental axioms that vital events cannot be regarded as summations, but always only from a unitary point of view.

CHAPTER VI

Understanding and explaining.—The attempt at sympathetic
  understanding of animal behaviour.—Intra-central orientation and disorientation of animals.—Comparative physiology
  of the senses and nerves in animal psychology.

In the biology of the last decade, a great part has been
played by the fiction that the living body is a machine,
and can be understood in its functions as we understand
a machine. We have set up against this the fiction that
the organism is something entirely different in nature
from inorganic matter. The difference between living and
non-living nature in the light of this view was discussed
at length in the first lecture. We will now assume further
that all other organisms are allied in nature to us human
beings, and to a greater degree, the nearer they are to us
in systematic classification. In this sense, therefore, the
plants and lower animals are very far removed from us :
but the further we rise in the zoological system, the
more similar do the animals, in a general way, become
to human beings in their nature.

When likenesses in nature exist, understanding is
possible. This brings me to the difference between
" understanding " and " explaining ". (I am using these
two terms in a somewhat different sense from the psychological school of Heidelberg.) Understanding is something primary, something which is set up directly, while
explaining is something secondary, in which the main

part is played by experience and rational consideration. I observe, for example, that a pair of birds fall, when I approach their nest, into very rapid motion, flutter around, and emit continual cries. I can attempt to grasp this process from two sides, either by striving to understand it by sympathy, or by attempting to explain it from the physiological processes taking place in the senses, nerves, and organs of motion of the two individual birds. It appears to me that sympathetic understanding is able to bring us into a more direct relation to the observed facts, and that explanation from physiological processes can play in this case only a more modest part.

On the other hand, my understanding fails me when I watch the same pair of birds building their nest. For in the case of ourselves, the construction of so complicated an affair is something that must be first learned by example; but the bird's power of building its nest is inborn, and when the time of pairing arrives, it builds the nest characteristic of its species, even when it itself was not brought up in such a nest, and has never in its life seen one. It is here that a limit is set to my understanding; if I attempt to assume that the bird possesses a psychical constitution analogous to my own, there is no inward resonance in my own mind which tells me what passes in the bird while it is building its nest. I have no alternative but to use my experience as a biologist to " explain " the whole process by saying that this particular power is inborn in this particular bird.

Of course, understanding and explaining are not crass opposites, and there are numerous cases in which understanding and explaining are both mingled as far as I am concerned. Such a case is when the duck mother leads her new-hatched children immediately to the water. The instinct to take care of offspring is one that I can understand through direct human experience; the fact that the female duck also has an inward compulsion to take its children to water is something that I cannot inwardly understand, but must explain from my general knowledge by saying that this is a characteristic of ducks and other aquatic birds.

Furthermore, even in the case of my fellow human beings I am not able to understand everything, but and in many cases compelled to limit myself to explaining behaviour which I observe. An unmusical person, for example, is entirely unable to put himself in the place of a musical person listening to a concert; he simply learns by experience that a certain musical person exhibits, on hearing a certain piece of music, an emotional reaction, while other pieces of music do not produce this effect. The same is true as regards the attitude, as observed by the unmusical person, of musically inclined people towards executants: one of the latter will be appreciated, while another will receive no applause. After a sufficient time, the unmusical person is able to foresee how a definite person, or number of persons, will react when such and such an artist plays a certain piece. But he will not understand this sympathetically, but simply be able to explain it on the basis of his previous experience.

The healthy person's power of understanding frequently fails him when confronted with the mentally ailing, and there remains only the method of explanation. In a situation the danger of which we recognize objectively, we are able to understand directly the expression of fear, but the healthy person fails to understand the behaviour of a person suffering from persecution mania for example, and he is obliged to accept the explanation of the psychiatrist, that in this disease the symptoms of persecution mania appear.

It is also evident that understanding and explanation are not irreconcilable opposites as regards the behaviour of our fellow-men. It may often occur that I understand an action to a large degree, but there remains to me a residue, which, in spite of my best efforts, can only be explained. In other cases, I may be dealing with behaviour which in the main I can only explain, nevertheless there may be some point where I can understand and sympathize.

It is only psychical processes—or more correctly their mode of expression—which can be understood; bodily functions such as the activity of the intestines or the heart, growth, etc., are always only susceptible of explanation. I believe this also to be true, even when we set up the fiction that these functions are the manifestation of a psyche-like agent working for the maintenance of the individual whole.

So much for the difference between understanding and explaining. We will now consider more fully to what extent we may dare to attempt to grasp the behaviour of animals by understanding. In the last chapter we spoke of animals which run directly either towards or away from a source of light. This behaviour is called positive and negative phototaxis. The animals themselves are described accordingly as photopositive and

E

photonegative; on account of their inner distribution, their photopositivity or photonegativity, we have them exhibiting positive or negative phototaxis. We take a photopositive animal—a crab or an insect—and vary the experiment already described by using, in a darkened laboratory, not one source of light, but two. The two lamps are of equal strength, the starting point is equally distant, and at the commencement of the experiment the animal sees them symmetrically. Several possibilities of behaviour then exist. The animal may run directly towards one lamp, without taking any notice of the other; or it may run for a space along the line midway between the two lamps, and decide later for one or the other; or it may move in a zig-zag for short distances first in the direction of one lamp and then of the other, its path finally ending at one of them. If we experiment with one and the same animal several times in succession, these various forms of track may appear in the most various fashion. According to the theory of tropotaxis, a photopositive animal reaches the lamp on that side from which its eyes are more strongly illuminated. If the animal, therefore, runs from the start towards one lamp, it is assumed that this lamp sent a stronger light to its eyes in the first place. If the animal moves a space along the midway direction, the light stimuli from right and left are supposed to be of equal strength, so that the animal, like a horse on two pairs of reins, is led along at an equal distance from the two sources of stimulus; the decision, as to the side to which it finally turns, is supposed to depend upon its eyes being more intensively illuminated by one lamp in the course of a " chance " turn. And the zig-zag course is supposed to be the result of more light falling " by chance " first from one side and then from the other upon the eyes of the experimental animal.

The theory of tropotaxis therefore degrades the animal to the level of a machine, which is directed by the rays of light hither and thither like a puppet on strings. As opposed to this fiction, that the behaviour of an animal is brought about as the sum of the opposed functions of the right and left side of the body, we have set up the fiction that the behaviour of the animal must always be regarded as a whole. According to this view, the animal therefore sees both lamps from the start. In one case, it decides straight away for one of them and leaves the other unnoticed ; it " fixates itself intra-centrally " upon one source of light, and, eliminates the other intra-centrally, as I have termed it. Or the animal postpones a decision, and moves for a space along the middle line, only deciding later to turn finally to one or other source of light. Or the animal " hesitates intra-centrally " between the two sources of stimulus ; the expression of this indecision is its zig-zag course, each change in its direction signifying a change in decision. While the theory of tropotaxis only explains the behaviour of the photopositive animal in the experiment with two lights, as due to the difference between the amount of light reaching the right-hand and the left-hand side of the body, I have attempted to understand by sympathy its behaviour in the manner stated above. According to the expression I have used, the animal " decides " either from .the start or after having moved a certain distance ; the animal is " undecided ", it " hesitates " between two objectives, and is able to " alter its decision ".

This kind of behaviour I observed in particular regarding the hermit crab (*Eupagurus*), with which I have made many experiments. All varieties of crab possess two pairs of feelers, and in the case of the hermit crab, the first pair is short and the second long. The latter pair are used for feeling, the first for chemically testing the water. This is effected by the crab beating the water rapidly with its first pair of feelers. It looks as if it were making signs in the Morse code. If the hermit crab sees any striking object, it is able to beat its feelers in that direction. The hermit crab does not move only, as do most other animals, symmetrically in the direction of its own axis, but it even more frequently moves in an oblique direction forwards or sideways towards its goal. This cannot be understood in the sense of the theories of tropism and tropotaxis, for when it is set obliquely to its path, the two eyes are unequally illuminated, and yet the animal arrives without deviation and along a straight path to the source of stimulus. The explanation is to be found in the fact that the reaction is that of the animal as a whole, and is not the result of the addition of the two halves of the body acting separately.

In the experiment with two lamps, the hermit crab either moves from the start in a straight line towards one of them, in which case it waves its first pair of feelers only towards this during its whole march. Or it may move for a space along the middle line between the lamps ; in this case it rapidly changes from waving towards one to waving towards the other ; this leads us to conclude that the animal observes both lamps separately, but that it postpones for a time a decision as to which it shall approach. It is also important that the crab can move along this middle line with its body in any kind of oblique relationship to it, and this means that the two eyes may be entirely differently illuminated. We get a zig-zag course when the animal decides as it moves along its path, first in favour of one and then in favour of the other. If we alter the position of the start, so that it is not equally distant from the two lamps, the intensity of light reaching it from the two is not equal. Quantities of light are indirectly proportional to the square of the distances ; if, for example, the distance to the one lamp is fifty centimetres, and to the other seventy, twice the amount of light reaches the crab from the first than from the second. Under these conditions, the hermit crab is able to decide from the start for either of the lamps ; hence it is by no means " drawn " in the sense of the theory of tropotaxis towards that lamp from which at the start it receives most light. When the crab has reached one of the lamps, it may immediately leave this and proceed to the other ; calculation shows that a lamp to which the crab is very close may be exposing it to a light one or two thousand times as strong as the other, nevertheless the crab leaves the one and runs towards the other. The animal is thus by no means " a slave of the light " or " of its sense organs ", but is able to choose quite independently of the circumstances of the experiment and make a decision.

I have also experimented with the shore crab (*Carcinus*). This animal always proves to be photonegative, that is, it never runs towards the light, but always avoids it. On the other hand, we are able to use, as objectives for it, black screens which were offered to experimental animals contained in a white vessel. These screens were five centimetres broad, about corresponding to the diameter of the individuals used. Exactly the same experiments could be done with these black screens on the photo-negative shore crab as were performed with lights on the photopositive Eupagurus. One point deserves special notice : lamps emit light, that is radiant energy, and this circumstance has led a number of upholders of the theories of tropism and tropotaxis to refer the resulting locomotion of an animal towards a light or away from it to a kind of transformation of energy ; according to this, the light energy is supposed to be transformed by means of the central nervous system into motor energy. But it is characteristic of black screens that they do not give out any kind of energy, nevertheless the motion of the shore crab is directed towards them. Hence the fact that an object serves as the goal of an animal is not decided by whether it emits energy, and how much energy it emits, but only by whether it can be distinguished from the surroundings by the animal.

In the case of the shore crab, we must distinguish two intra-central dispositions ; one to running around, and another to seeking a point of rest. In the case of the first the animal runs only in the general direction of a black screen offered to it, but then runs past it and around in the experimental vessel ; but when it was disposed to rest the crab runs straight to the screen and remains at it.

In the case of animals disposed to rest, it was possible to carry out experiments in the way we have indicated, and they were to correspond entirely with the light experiments on hermit crabs. In the presence of a black screen, the crab made for it straight from the start, though its body might be pointing in any direction ; in the course of its movement its first pair of feelers beat rapidly in the direction of the goal. If two screens were set up, the animal might run towards one of them, the other being completely ignored—intra-centrally eliminated. Or the crab ran for a space along the middle line, thus postponing the decision as to which screen it was to aim at ; its intra-central hesitation between the two goals was expressed by the fact that it waved its first feelers alternatively in the direction of one of the screens and of the other. Its course along the middle line could also be zig-zag ; the animal ran alternately towards the right and left screen, finishing up at one or the other. It is of importance tha t all its movements, both in the case of one screen and of two, could be carried out with its body in any direction, that is, symmetrically forwards, sideways, obliquely forwards, and even for a space, obliquely sideways or symmetrically backwards. And even on one and the same run, it might change its orientation several times.

I already took the opportunity in the first chapter to stress the fact that, in the case of the hermit and shore crabs when making straight for a goal, the orientation of their bodies with reference to their line of movement is of no importance. But this appears to me to demonstrate most impressively the " wholeness " of their behaviour. For at every change in the direction of the body other parts of the eyes perceive the goal, and each time the legs must move in a different manner, without any detriment to the directness of the motion towards the goal. For what decides the mode of locomotion is the intra-central fixation of the animal upon the goal; and according to the detailed nature of the situation at any moment, the " means " used to reach this goal are varied—in full agreement with the fictional axiom which we set up in the first chapter, that the end determines the means.

In discussions of the tropism and tropotaxis theories, a great part has been played by the behaviour of individuals blinded on one side in the experiments with single lights. In these cases, a photopositive animal so treated deviates towards the seeing side, a photonegative animal towards its blind side. This is explained by the tropism and tropotaxis theories by saying that the artificial asymmetry of the light receptors (the eyes) results in the muscles of motion receiving asymmetrical impulses, and this unequal functioning of the two sides of the body is supposed to result in a deviation towards that side acting less strongly.

We reject this view, and shall attempt to get nearer to the process by an understanding of it. We take a crab or an insect and blind it on one side. This can be done in two ways: either by coating the eye with an opaque black varnish, or by removing it. The effect is the same: the animal now only sees on one side, and is hence easily deceived as to the state of illumination of its surroundings; it can thus be deluded that brightness exists only on its seeing side, and that its blind side is dark. According as we are dealing with a photopositive or photonegative animal, its behaviour is different; the photopositive animal turns towards the seeing side, the photonegative animal towards the blind side. This is the interpretations which has been given by V. Buddenbrock and myself as regards the behaviour of animals blinded on one side. If we hesitate to make use of the word " delusion " as regards an animal, we may say that the injury has " intra-centrally disorientated " the blinded animal as regards the stimulus situation. I have distinguished between the bodily orientation of animals in space, and their intra-central orientation concerning the peculiarities of the medium. According to the degree of its adjustment, an animal takes up a more or less correct orientation in space corresponding to the situation, and if it is completely disadjusted intra-centrally, behaviour out of correspondence with the situation results.

The concepts of intra-central adjustment and disadjustment are fictions, which the experimenter is able to abstract from his observations. He knows that in such and such a situation the members of a species behave in such a way ; an intact photopositive animal, for example, makes straight for the light, while a photonegative animal makes straight away from it ; if an animal blinded on one side wanders, it is wanting, in the view we have put forward, with respect to intra-central adjustment of the situation. If we test the behaviour of an animal blinded on one side in detail, we observe that adjustment and disadjustment frequently alternate rapidly. Sometimes the animal will attain or avoid the lamp by a straight line movement, at another time it will wander. A change of this kind may even take place during one and the same run, that is, at times the animal succeeds with the aid of its one uninjured eye, in adjusting itself to the distribution of stimulus in its surroundings, but again falls into delusion due to being blind on one side. In the case of the photonegative shore crab, blinding and a black screen may compete with one another; in this case the animal runs at one time towards the screen, and at another towards its blind side.

In certain circumstances the degree of adjustment may gradually improve in course of the experiment; Urban was able to demonstrate this by experiments on bees carried out in the Zoological Institute at Marburg. Immediately after blinding, the photopositive animals ran in close spirals towards the seeing side, and thus only moved quite gradually towards the light. But the spirals gradually became longer, until the paths became straight. Temporary relapses into the original disadjustment might occur; that is to say, from time to time a single spiral movement might take place.

At the close of this chapter it appears to me advisable to define the limits between the comparative physiology of the senses and nerves, on the one hand, and animal psychology on the other. Hitherto these two terms have often been confused, so that in the case of many authors, matter belonging to the physiology of the senses was already regarded as ranking under animal psychology. Comparative physiology is concerned quite generally with the manner of functioning of single organs, that is to say, of the sense organs, the central nervous system, and the effectors (for example, the muscles, glands, etc.). Or it investigates single processes, such as walking, flying, standing upright, digestion, and the like. Very frequently, the single organs cannot be completely separated for the purpose of investigation, from the rest of the body, but must be left in connection with it. The physiology of the senses and nerves then studies what the animal does in the presence and in the absence of a certain sense organ or part of the central nervous system. As long as a certain stereotyped character of behaviour results, and as long as it can be proved that the varying results are determined from outside—by artificial changes in the organs or by alteration in the experimental arrangement —we are dealing with physiology of the senses or nerves respectively. But as soon as the course of events varies in a manner which points away from such direct connections with external factors, and suggests factors of an internal nature, the task of animal psychology commences. Hence, comparative physiology of the senses and nerves is rather a study of partial processes, while that of animal psychology is a study of the behaviour of the whole, the main attention being directed towards variations produced purely intra-centrally.

CHAPTER VII

The animal's grasp of wholes.—Super-individual wholes.

WITH the aid of our eyes we recognize a human being as such whether he is in our immediate neighbourhood or a certain distance away. His actually apparent size is of no importance for us ; furthermore, in the process of recognition, no part is played by the bodily position of the person recognized, or by our own. A man thus remains a man for us, whether he is standing or sitting before our eyes, so that we either see his right or left side, his front or his back, or watch him lying down, walking, running and so on. And, as we have said, the same is true for ourselves as observers ; whether we are at rest or in motion, and in whatever way, we always recognize in the same manner. Again, the most various types of human beings are immediately recognized by us for what they are, whatever may be their appearance and form in detail. We conclude from all this that recognition does not depend so much upon how many, and which, of the elements of vision are excited on our retina. Our eye is only the organ of reception, which transmits the stimuli received to our central nervous system. The act of recognition is a purely intra-central event, and this recognition does not merely occur when what is recognized corresponds to a single or a few types, but on the contrary, there are unlimited possibilities in the ways in which optical impressions of an external object, for example a human being, can reach us, and none the less, the person in question is immediately and directly recognized by us as a human being. The process of recognition, therefore, never takes place in any schematic and automatic way, but always bears entirely a creative character.

In the same way as we immediately recognize a person unknown to us as a human being, we also recognize the identity of someone known to us, whatever the external situation. He is, whatever the orientation in space, directly and undoubtedly one and the same. His picture for us has been completed by bodily movements, which we call " characteristics ", without their ever being carried out in exactly the same manner, and by his voice, although he scarcely ever says exactly the same thing, and by many other peculiarities. And in the same way, a table is for us a table, a tree a tree, a horse a horse, a triangle a triangle, without regard to the individual peculiarities of these objects, and their momentary arrangement and position. Here is a problem, which we generally overlook, since the facts just referred to are extremely familiar to us in our daily life, and hence appear self-evident. According to the point of view we are taking, this phenomenon must be regarded as follows : The recognition of an object or a certain person by ourselves does not take place additively from the sum of single peculiarities observed, but as a whole (in the terms used by W. Koehler and Wertheimer, as a *Gestalt*). I first grasp, therefore, the whole (the *Gestalt*) of the object presented to me, and only thereupon do I perceive a greater or less number of single data, according to the degree in which I turn my attention to them. In the same way, I am myself, as object of my own observation, always in the first place an undivided whole, which is not originally, but only after a process of laborious intellectual analysis, perceived to be made up of a sum of single data.

We will now enquire whether our consideration of the subject will be furthered by the fiction that not only man, but also an animal, grasps itself and the objects of its surroundings as wholes. We take a spider's web, and destroy a part of it. If we do serious damage, the spider abandons the web; but if the damage is less serious it mends the injured part by drawing new threads in a manner adapted to the situation. It appears to me that we must here speak of the spider grasping the matter as a whole. For before we do the damage, it has produced a whole: its web. It recognizes, when we injure it, whether repair is worth while or not; in the first case it restores the damaged whole by addition of the required threads. We are not able to understand its intra-central situation, from which its sureness is derived without previous example and learning; we do not know whether the animal is conscious during the processes of spinning and repair at all, or if so, of what it is conscious. We have already seen that the question of animal conscious-ness cannot be attacked by scientific methods; but even if the contents of the consciousness of animals, in this case of a spider, were known to us, we should not be much further advanced. For even in the case of human beings, the deep psychology founded upon the doctrines of Freud, Adler, Jung, Stekel, and others, has shown us that the contents of consciousness are often of least importance in deciding action ; much greater importance usually attaches to what exists on the other side—as it were—behind the conscious personality.

Just as, in our own case, our grasp of wholes comes out of unknown depths, just as it is given to us with compulsive necessity from the structure of our brain and intellectual organization, so also is the grasp by the spider of a whole inseparably linked with its whole nature. That so highly specialized a grasp of wholes should exist in an inborn form, without having been individually acquired, appears to us human beings extraordinarily strange. We are not able to understand it on the basis of our own organization, but are obliged to be content with simply registering the phenomenon.

The animal also recognizes other members of its species as wholes, in so far as it comes into relation with them. Thus, for the animal—as for man—the sexual partner, for example, is not a conglomerate of single data, but a complete whole, the parts of which must be put together in a certain way and not otherwise.

The *Gestalt* of the partner requires in some cases, to comprise not only a certain optical impression, but also a voice or peculiar smell, which plays a great part in the case of many animals. Stimuli produced by contact may also be of importance.

The first alarm which the animal receives of the presence in its neighbourhood of an enemy, a prey, or a sexual partner, may be given by single data of one of the senses : hearing, sight, smell, or touch ; on the other hand, the

way the new arrival is dealt with, the defence against
the enemy, the attack on the prey, the act of copulation,
is always a matter of the whole. There are certain kinds
of animals which are wanting in one of the senses named,
for example hearing or sight; but this by no means
detracts from the wholeness of their reaction. The same
is true of the blind or deaf human being. A blind man
can only gradually form a conception of the shape of
a body by feeling it; nevertheless, in spite of the fact
that the tactual impressions are only acquired gradually,
the final result is a conception of the whole body. For
it is of no importance as regards the grasp of a whole,
whether the sense data concerned are received simultaneously, or one after another; this is true, for example,
of the spider, which does not take in its whole web at
a single glance, but runs all over it and thus notices a
certain defect. The case of the blind man is similar:
he forms the impression of a body as a whole out of a
set of separate tactual impressions.

There is even no obstacle to the fiction that the animal
grasps itself as a whole, and it allows us to do justice to
the fact that the activities of animals always bear the
character of wholeness. Of course, we are not maintaining
that the animal is conscious of itself as a whole; the
matter of consciousness, as we have seen, has very little
point in this connection. Deep psychology has taught
us that the behaviour of a fellow human-being can be
much more comprehensively grasped when we lay
less stress upon what takes place in his consciousness,
but rather neglect this to a great extent. When
attempting to understand the behaviour of animals,

we may leave the question of consciousness entirely aside.

We set up the fiction that the hermit crab, for example, which in moving straight towards a lamp, turns its body now one way and now another in quite an irregular manner, is for itself, and to itself, a whole. Its body is the instrument which serves to reach its goal; it performs motion in a straight line while handling this instrument in the most various manner. Another example; a bird striving towards a goal by swimming, flying, and running in turn, is itself a whole; it is able to vary the means from one moment to another, while its action is determined by the goal.

In the foregoing we have imagined that we are able to understand the behaviour of an animal by sympathy. Here we are taking no account of the question whether the animal possesses consciousness and understands itself. In order to discuss this assertion more fully we must return to the question of how understanding takes place among human beings. One human being can very well understand another, without the latter understanding himself. This kind of understanding plays a great part in more recent psycho-therapy and teaching; thus the doctor, for example, may make clear to the patient the purpose of his neurosis, of which he has hitherto been ignorant. In many cases, therefore, the content of the consciousness of the person to be understood has in the first place nothing to do with the matter.

We must, however, remember that understanding is a completely subjective phenomenon; hence, several persons forming a judgment may, according to various

F

circumstances, understand and experience sympathetically one and the same person from different points of view, each depending also upon the inward situation of its possessor ; for every observer is dependent, as regards what seems important to him, almost entirely upon his own psychical organization. Thus the nature and character of understanding result not only from the nature of the being to be understood, but also from that of the one understanding ; we need in no way assume misunderstanding, when one observer regards and experiences sympathetically the behaviour of a person more in one way, and another more in another way.

Furthermore, one person may understand another in the deeper sense, even when he is by no means clearly conscious of all the details of the latter's behaviour ; in fact, understanding is not in itself so much a matter of what is present in the consciousness of the subject. This allows us to suppose that an animal, also, is able to understand the behaviour of another animal, or that of a human being ; and in this case, according to what we have just said, there is for the moment no need to take further into account what takes place, during the process, in the first animal's consciousness.

With this, the concepts of understanding and of being able to understand have acquired a fictional character ; the importance of this fiction lies in our being able, with its aid, to assert that human beings can directly understand animals, and that these may understand, on the one hand one another, and on the other hand human beings, though only within certain limits.

By way of conclusion, we will once more consider the

question whether wholes exist which extend beyond single individuals—super-individual wholes, as we may call them, of which the single individual forms only a part. When we observe various species of animals and plants in their natural surroundings, we see that they are adapted to these in the completest manner. We owe to von Uexküll very profound observations in this direction. According to this author, each species of animal selects from its surroundings what is biologically important for it, and capable of being grasped by its sense organs; only this is " environment ", or " the surrounding world " for it. And each species of animal therefore lives in its surroundings in a glass case, as it were. In the world of earthworms, there are only " earthworm things " ; in that of the dragonfly, " dragonfly things " ; in that of the dog, only " dog things ". If therefore two animals belonging to different species are in the same place, their relative environments may be completely different. The same is evidently true for human beings, where great differentiation exists according to race, social position, age, occupation, etc. It is well known " with what different eyes " a landscape, for example, is seen by a painter, a geologist, or a strategist ; for each of these men, quite different features of the terrain are important and unimportant.

Legewie has pointed out that for one and the same individual animal, the surrounding world can be entirely different according to the physiological conditions in which it finds itself ; thus the hungry animal has quite a different surrounding world from that of the satisfied creature, the animal before copulation a different one

from afterwards, etc. According to the inward physiological situation, various objects of the surroundings and
of the surrounding world assume importance from time
to time. The same thing is true of man ; not only in the
course of his individual development, as child, adult,
and in old age, does he form from the total environment
quite different subjective surrounding worlds ; even at
one and the same stage of development—even from hour
to hour—various things assume great importance at one
time, while at another they are completely unnoticed.
In and out of the daily occupation, before and after
meals, before and after sleep, in sickness and in health,
the " surrounding world " has an altogether different
constitution.

Are we then to describe the organism and its total
environment, or such living and non-living things as it
takes from the latter as important—the organism therefore
and its relative surrounding world—as a super-individual
whole ? Whether such a fiction proves useful or not,
depends upon the special scientific purpose which we
are pursuing. In the present case it does not seem to me
correct to take this course ; the concept of super-
individual wholes should be defined more narrowly when
we are considering questions of animal psychology. For
the organism is adjusted in the most exact manner to its
environment, and fitted to live in it ; while the converse
of this cannot be asserted. The environment in which
we find organisms is constituted without any reference
to the latter. The various positions therefore, in which
animals and plants make their homes, the rocky cliff,
the sea-coast, the prairie, and other localities, are for the

most part pure aggregations of certain characteristics, and not wholes in the very narrow sense in which we are using the word at present; the reader may be referred in this connection to the first chapter. It is true that the individual animal grasps its environment as a whole, and deals with it in a unitary manner; but I do not feel justified in regarding such relationships between the organism and its environment as resulting in the formation of a super-individual whole. Hence we shall not apply this notion in all cases where the organism is, as it were, one partner, and the environmental aggregate of living and non-living elements, or that relative environment abstracted from it, the other partner. We shall only speak of a super-individual whole when two or more living organisms enter into relationship with one another. But not every form of such association is sufficient to produce a whole; when animals meet at the same feeding place (for example, flies on a piece of carrion, cattle at a watering-place, etc.), this chance collection (conglobation, see Chapter X) is by no means enough to form a super-individual whole. In the same way, the struggle between an animal and its prey, or between two beasts of prey, does not result in the formation of a whole.

We shall confine the notion of super-individual wholes to those cases where the individuals show themselves during a relationship (which furthermore must not last for too short a time), to be linked to one another inwardly. Super-individual wholes in this sense are to be regarded as embodied in animal matings, animal families and animal societies, with which we shall deal more in detail in Chapter X. To go beyond this, and to apply the fiction of the super-individual whole to all individuals belonging to one and the same species, is not a necessity in the present connection.   A species might, however, be regarded as a closed procreative community of all its individuals, and thus be defined as a super-individual whole ; but we will not here make use of this possibility, but merely refer to it.

CHAPTER VIII

Primary and secondary knowledge.—Instinctive and experiential activity.

WE have already discussed at an earlier stage an important difference between man and animals, the difference, namely, that in many cases animals possess innately faculties which man must acquirel aboriously. Many animals are able to run or swim from their birth; the spider spins its web without example or practice, the bird makes its nest, when the time comes, without ever having seen such a nest before. The caterpillars of many species of butterflies spin a cocoon shortly before the pupa stage; and this may have special arrangements which later aid the butterfly in creeping out. Examples of this kind can be multiplied indefinitely; they all have this in common, that the animals in question are able to exercise a certain activity without example and without learning, and in a perfect manner.

In such cases, therefore, we are not dealing with aptitudes for activity which have been individually acquired, but with those which have been inherited; at a given time—sometimes directly after birth, sometimes in the course of later life—the animal proceeds to exhibit behaviour characteristic of its species. The term instinct has been applied to this; a notion which has been the subject of much controversy. Many authors have demanded that it should be eliminated entirely as being too "mystical". When, in the following pages, we speak of instinct, the reader is to understand nothing more by the term than an inherited aptitude for an activity; instinct shall be a symbolic term for a power hidden in the animal and manifested by it at a given moment.

We will take as synonymous with the notion of instinct that of the drive; whoever desires to avoid the first word, may use the second. An activity set going by an instinct or drive is an instinctive or drive activity; it is contrasted with experiential activity, which is brought about by practice and learning. Such experiential activities play, as we know, by far the greater part in human life; practically nothing in the behaviour of the adult human being is inborn; he is obliged to learn almost everything.

If we describe knowledge acquired by practice and experience as *secondary*, we may call the inherited aptitude for activity *primary* knowledge. The question as to whether or how far consciousness accompanies the utilization of primary or secondary knowledge is here pointless. We know from ourselves that there are actions which, once learned, we are finally able to execute without the need for our conscious attention. Walking and bicycling may be carried on without our consciousness having any part in their details. Our daily walk to our occupation, the winding of a watch, even the writing of the address on an envelope or the posting of the letter—all these are actions which, after they have been many times repeated, may be accompanied by so small a degree of conscious attention to them, that we may often be afterwards at a loss to remember whether or how we performed them.

We will now enquire whether man possesses only secondary or acquired knowledge, or whether he may possess inherited aptitudes to activity, however narrow their limits may be. The new-born human being brings with him into the world the capacity for sucking and swallowing. This is something that he does not need to learn, but is able to execute from the first. Here we are therefore dealing with an inborn or primary knowledge, an instinct in our sense of the term, whereby we leave entirely out of consideration the extent to which the infant is consciously aware of itself and of its own action. Furthermore, the new-born infant possesses a peculiar grip reaction—obviously an ancient inheritance, which has largely lost its importance for present-day man. For our ancestors, this reaction was most certainly of importance, as it still is for apes today, for it leads to the infant taking firm hold of its mother.

An inherited aptitude to activity, which is first manifested in man in the course of his development, is that for sexual action and its preliminaries; here we have a drive which gradually becomes more and more pronounced, an instinct, which leads to action of a quite definite character. Some authors have summarily declared instinctive actions to be unconscious; but the last-mentioned example of a typical instinctive action in the case of man, shows without further question that " unconscious " and " instinctive " are not to be regarded as equivalent; for no one will maintain that human action in sexual matters takes place without participation of consciousness. But in other respects, inherited aptitude to activity is practically completely absent in the case of man; but on the other hand, he has received a strong drive to accumulate secondary knowledge. The young child finds itself, as it were, in the position of an explorer who has landed upon a hitherto undiscovered island, and now finds everything, both as regards land and inhabitants, completely unknown and worthy of investigation. As the child's bodily development progresses, its mental horizon extends; while its environment is at first almost without detail, it becomes, in course of time, continually more differentiated and rich. But in this process the child's grasp of its surroundings never proceeds by mere aggregation, but always as a whole: the world is first present to it as an undifferentiated whole, and only gradually do more and more numerous details begin to become prominent. Also, in all that the child learns by its own powers and efforts, the whole is present before the parts, as for example in learning to speak. At a certain age the child produces a series of sounds, which have similarity with sentences, but are entirely un-articulated; primordial sentences, as I may call them. From these, sentences correct from the adult's point of view are gradually differentiated; this process might be compared with the development of the complete individual from the embryo. The egg and the embryo are not merely a sum of single parts, but whole structures at every stage; here, also, the whole is first present; the ovum and later the embryo; from these the parts, that is, the organs, are differentiated step by step.

In contrast to mankind, animals possess many inborn

aptitudes; these form their primary knowledge. We may now ask whether or to what extent animals are also capable of acquiring secondary knowledge, and to what extent, therefore, they are able to acquire experience. We easily succeed in training both higher and lower animals in such a way that a biologically indifferent stimulus becomes associated in them with a biologically important one; if the two stimuli are frequently allowed to operate simultaneously, they are linked together in the animal intra-centrally, in such a way that it finally reacts when only the biologically indifferent stimulus is given to it, which stimulus before training did not cause a reaction. The biologically important stimulus is called unconditioned, since it always and invariably produces a reaction; the biologically indifferent is called the conditioned stimulus, since it is only responded to conditionally, that is to say, after successful training.

Bees can be trained to respond to certain colours, blue or yellow; for example, they are given for a period their food, say sugar and water, upon a blue surface; this finally leads to the individuals in question alighting upon every blue surface, whether food is present upon it or not. In the same way fish can be brought to visit only a vessel of a certain colour, for example, red, all other food vessels of different colour being ignored. It is necessary in this case to offer the experimental animal simultaneously a number of small vessels of different colours, and repeat this several times, whereby food is always contained only in one, namely, the red vessel. Fish may also be trained for sound; if they are frequently fed while a sound of a certain pitch is given simultaneously, they finally swim up when they hear this " food note ", although there may be no food awaiting them. The number of cases in which animals can be trained to respond to biologically indifferent stimuli can be extended indefinitely. The cases of the bees and fish just mentioned were positive training, that is to say the experimental animal first reacted to the unconditioned, and then also to the conditioned stimulus, positively, by moving towards it. By way of contrast we have negative training, in which the experimental animal answers negatively, when the stimulus is offered, by moving away. We allow an earthworm to creep several times into the vertical limb of a T-shaped glass tube, when it reaches the two side arms it decides with equal frequency to go to the right or the left, as long as similar conditions exist on the two sides. We then close one arm, for example the left, to the animal, by introducing an electric circuit, so that the animal receives a shock every time it creeps into this tube. The earthworm very soon learns to avoid the left arm, and only passes into the right one. Similar negative training can be carried out on many other animals ; an indifferent stimulus is always associated as the conditional stimulus with a punishment stimulus as the unconditional. Thus, for example, the cockroach will learn, like the earthworm, to move right or left to avoid punishment, in frogs a punishment reaction can be associated with certain colours, and so on. In other words, it is easy to prove under the simplified and clear conditions which can be set up in the laboratory that animals of the most various systematic groups are able to learn, that is to say, acquire secondary knowledge.

We find that in natural conditions also, animals store up secondary knowledge and make use of it in their later behaviour. Bees, ants, and other insects learn by experience to know the surroundings of their nests, so that they can find their way back from every direction. On the rocky coasts of various seas there lives, in the tidal region, the common limpet (*Patella*). Each individual of this species returns at every ebb tide to the same place, where it remains until the sea returns. At the flood tide it feeds upon the small algae of the surrounding rocks and then returns in good time—from any direction whatsoever—to its accustomed resting-place. It finds the way by reference to the peculiarities of its surroundings; if with a hammer and chisel the surface of the rock is changed, the animal is no longer able to find its old resting-place.

In other ways also, many animals are able to learn: they remember the place at which they have frequently found food. Particularly higher animals, such as birds and mammals, know exactly the spots at which they are harried, and where they are safe. Furthermore, ravens, for example, are able to distinguish a sportsman from harmless pedestrians; deer have become assured of the innocuousness of the trains that thunder past, so that when grazing they do not show the slightest signs of disturbance, whereas the approach of a single person will put them to flight. Higher animals kept in captivity distinguish their keepers from other people: sometimes they will only take their food from the former. We could bring innumerable other examples to show that in the life of animals, their individual and acquired experience plays a part alongside their inherited aptitude for certain activities.

It has already been pointed out that we, from our human standpoint, are not able to enter into the inward situation of an animal which carries out, by inherited aptitude, some kind of complicated activity ; for example, that of the spider, when spinning its web or repairing it when defective. Power of this kind is almost miraculous to us. In such cases recourse has been had to the idea of instinct ; on certain sides something supernatural has actually been supposed to be at the back of instinct, and hence from other sides it has been looked upon with great disfavour. But let us consider a moment : is an inherited aptitude for an activity something more wonderful than the morphological structure of an animal's body and the interaction of the physiological processes taking place in it ? Are, let us say, the conception and development of the individual, and the continuation of its bodily functions, already " explained by science ", and only the inherited aptitude still " unexplained " ? By no means. All that I have just named are phenomena which refuse to yield up their inward nature to our comprehension : they are one and all equally well " known " to us or also equally " unknown "—both expressions are equally applicable in this context. The animal that possesses an inherited aptitude has not only inherited its various organs, but also instructions, as it were, for the use of them ; thus equipped, it has no need for trial and experience, but knows what to do from the very beginning.

Finally, the following further question arises : is the presence of primary knowledge more wonderful than the power of man and animals to acquire secondary knowledge and to store it up ?   Here again, the answer is in the negative.   For are we able to state in the least degree what happens, " how we do it ", when we learn something ? If the instinctive actions of animals appear particularly wonderful to us, the reason is to be found in the fact that in our own behaviour instinct plays a very small part ; what we ourselves are accustomed to is the inherited organization and functioning of our own bodies, and the power of collecting experiences.   Nevertheless, all this is by no means " better known " to us, as regards its nature and origin, than any inherited aptitude for activity. For a very simple reason : all knowledge of this kind exceeds our human capacity and our power of comprehension by far, not only now and today, but for all future time.

Hitherto I have set primary and secondary knowledge, or action from instinct and action from experience, alongside one another ; and it might thus be imagined that these notions are to be taken as the expression of irreconcilable contrasts.   We will now enquire whether— either in the case of animals or man—activities exist in which instinctive and experiential elements are both concerned.   Let us return to the example of the power of bees and ants to return home : the instinctive drive is the impulse to swarm out, to learn by heart the surroundings of the nest, and then to return after each excursion ; at each excursion and each return, however, individual experience must play a part, inasmuch as the animal is compelled to keep in memory the details of its surroundings.   The primary part, therefore, is the knowledge that the nest must be left and then returned to again, while the details of the way in which this is to be effected are secondary knowledge. Furthermore, instinct and experience are mingled in all training ; the search for, and consumption of, food depend in themselves upon primary knowledge, and are inherited aptitudes ; but when the experimenter succeeds in training an animal to seek its food at a definite place or on a definite colour, experience is concerned in this behaviour as an important element.

In the various races of animals, the instinctive aptitudes are modifiable in varying degrees ; the instincts—as it has been expressed—are " plastic " to a variable extent. There are instincts possessing great rigidity. A frequently quoted case in this connection is that of a bee (*Chalicodoma*) which lives solitarily. The female builds a number of combs, charges each with a definite quantity of honey, lays an egg in it, and closes it up. If we bore a hole in a comb while the female is engaged in filling it with honey, it investigates, it is true, the hole and the escaping honey, but does not repair the damage, but proceeds to bring to the comb the remaining quantity of honey, to lay its egg there, and to close the comb, without reference to the fact that the honey is flowing away. Here we see that the limits of a highly complicated parental instinct can be drawn very narrowly ; we might suppose that the female would repair the injured comb immediately, since its bodily constitution renders it perfectly capable of doing so. But its central nervous organization is not prepared for this activity. The series : building the comb, bringing a measured quantity of honey, laying an egg, and covering up the comb, is adhered to with absolute rigidity, with complete indifference to the fact—visible to an observer—that the continuation of the series of activities has been rendered senseless by a disturbing element from outside.

We have already mentioned as an inherited aptitude that of the bird for building its nest. At a certain time, namely at the beginning of pairing, the bird builds a nest in accordance with its species, even when it has not itself been hatched out in such a nest, and has never seen one. But experience may also play a certain part in nest building, in so far as an older bird which has already built several nests will do so with greater skill than a young one.

The drive of the male bird to sing is inherited, and even when the young male has never heard the song of another bird, it commences at a given time to sing on its own account. But such an animal remains a poor performer ; and those males produce the most perfect song which have had an especially good example in an elder individual of their species. This is well known to breeders of canaries, chaffinches, nightingales and so on, and these give the birds they breed the best singers as teachers. Hence on the basis of a drive primarily present, that of singing, the form of the song in individual cases is determined by example and practice. It thus happens, for example, that finches in various parts sing differently ; they have, as it were, in each case adopted the dialect of the neighbourhood. Mockingbirds are able to learn the song of various species of birds and also to imitate other noises, such as the

G

creaking of cart wheels. In other species, on the other hand, the young male under natural conditions always seeks out an elder male of its species as a teacher; what is therefore primary in his case is the knowledge as to what kind of song he is to choose as an example, and on this basis he builds up his own powers as secondary knowledge.

Care of the offspring is an inherited aptitude in the case of many higher animals; it corresponds to the pairing instinct of young individuals. These two drives are plastic to a large degree; hence, if we take a young bird or a young mammal away from the parents or the mother immediately after birth, and give it as a fosterchild to an individual of another species, it continues to follow the latter, and later no longer recognizes its own parents. Hence in this case there is no " call of the blood ", any more than in the case of human beings. For the young bird, the human hand can take the place of the mother or the parents; if the young creature has been accustomed to it, it will seek refuge in the hand and avoid the parents. What is born therefore in the young bird or the young mammal is the need for protection; but this attaches itself differently, and to different objects, from case to case.

The instinct of the parents to care for the offspring is also plastic. Lloyd Morgan describes an extreme example. A hen three times hatched out young ducks. While on the first occasion it was somewhat upset when the young ducks immediately took to the water, it gradually became accustomed to this process with the second and third brood. A fourth brood consisted of her own offspring;

when these were hatched, the hen tried in all kinds of ways to persuade the young animals to enter the water, and even to drive them into it. In this case the normal instinct had become very greatly changed by habit.

CHAPTER IX

Instinct and experience in human beings.—Behaviour indicating insight in man and animals.

IT was shown in the last chapter that in human beings instinctive activities play a very small part as compared with those based upon experience. We mentioned sucking and swallowing in new-born children, and also their clutching reaction, as an example of inherited aptitude for activity; at puberty, the sex drive appears in a sharply defined form, after having already signalized its presence at an earlier age by various actions of a more diffused character.

It was shown in the last chapter that, in the case of animals, actions based on instinct and on experience are not to be regarded as opposite in nature, since the two extremes are connected by numerous intermediate stages, in which the purely instinctive element, and that dependent upon experience, are both concerned in bringing about a certain activity. Let us now see how the matter stands in the case of man. When a child learns to talk, and to get into contact with its surroundings in other ways as well, what is primary in this activity is the inherited drive. The gradual accustoming of the child to its environment is only successful on this basis. If the social instinct is defective or perverse in its development, the individual in question is the victim of an endless chain of very difficult external and internal conflicts. We thus see that the child must bring with it into the world a certain general readiness to adapt itself more and more to the world as that world is constituted. In this case, however, it is not a matter of specialized inherited aptitude for activity, such as we find in animals, but simply the aptitude of its species to assimilate those experiences which are necessary for its existence. But, as we all know, experience alone is not by any means sufficient for life ; behind this experience must exist the drive to activity and to making use of experience in practice. This drive to act and to take part in active life, is something primary ; the secondary stored-up knowledge is simply a means of finding one's place in the world and behaving in a manner suited to the immediate situation. Hence, in every action which we perform upon the basis of our experience, there is a component founded upon instinctive drive ; and great individual differences exist—it is a " matter of temperament " as we say—in the way in which experiences are made use of.

Activities in which, even in the case of adults, the drive component is immediately evident, are the absorption of nourishment and the sexual act. But even in these, secondary knowledge plays a part. There are very great variations as between one race, and one grade of society, and another, in the matter of when and what is eaten, and what is rejected ; and even in the sexual act, the importance of experience and custom cannot be denied.

A higher rank still must be assigned to actions based upon insight, than upon those based upon experience. What is common in these two forms of behaviour is plasticity, but whereas in the case of experiential activity, there is a previous stage of trial, practice, or learning, it is characteristic of behaviour based upon insight— apart from a short period of latency which may occur— that there is a lightning-like grasp and comprehension of the situation. Experiential action and action based upon insight, are not opposites, for the latter may be regarded as experiential action of a very shortened character. Observation of ourselves teaches us how numerous are the intermediate stages between activities which can only be exercised after long trial and practice, such actions as depend upon the solution of a problem being perceived by us directly. The intermediate stages are formed by activities which are preceded only by a short period of trial, or in which the period of trial becomes transferred to a mental process ; and we are also no doubt justified in assuming that, in all behaviour based upon insight, earlier experience of some kind plays a part.

It must further be said that any behaviour in which a complete solution is not arrived at also frequently depends upon insight. For the word " insight " is not used in the sense of a judgment of values, but merely to characterize a certain type of behaviour in which the outside world has to be dealt with. We each know from our own experience that there are innumerable stages between insight which immediately leads to a true solution of a problem, and complete want of understanding of a situation. Matters are further complicated by the fact that between the observer and the person observed there may be a difference of opinion as to whether a complete solution of a problem has been obtained or not ; the person observed may be subjectively of the opinion that the problem was solved ; whereas the observer may maintain that it was only partially solved. All conceptual difficulties of this kind disappear when we require as the criterion of insight, not insight in a valuable sense, but only a certain form of prompt reaction, which allows of complete solution and also of partial solution.

It would be completely erroneous to contrast activities based upon experience or insight with instinctive actions by calling them " voluntary actions ", for our will also takes part in setting in motion drive actions such as feeding or copulation ; the organs in question send signals to our brain, and the will impulse then results accordingly. How the will is formed in special cases of this and similar character is completely impenetrable, and must always remain so. Whether our will is in any sense " free " (in the sense of indeterminate) cannot be decided. We are subjectively of the opinion that we act freely after conscious consideration of all motives, when, for example, we decide whether we shall go to a concert or not ; or we may believe that a writer has complete and conscious freedom as to whether he will have one of the characters in a play die or not. Recent medical psychology maintains, however, another opinion (see for example, Kretschmer). According to this school of thought, the motives which determine whether, to take our example, we visit a concert or stay at home, may never reach our consciousness at all ; and when the writer works out his play, nothing in it is freely formed, or even a matter of chance, but on the contrary, the whole work and all its parts are definite and unambiguous forms of expression of its author's whole psychical make-up.

We know nothing of the part played by consciousness in our own psychical processes. It certainly plays a part in those activities which we describe as our " highest " ; in trial, practice, learning, consideration, and in the attainment of insight and so on. But how we manage to arrive at a certain insight, how we try out something or learn something, and how we put our experience into practice, are matters which we cannot describe. We have too strong a tendency to experience everything taking place in consciousness as constituting our " self ", and to ignore the unconscious. But without the latter, consciousness could not exist at all ; it would be entirely without any root and foundation. In the case of man there are experiential activities which must first of all be learned and practised consciously, and can then be carried out without consciousness playing any part in them ; I refer to cycling, winding up a watch, etc. Actions of this kind are called " acquired automatisms ". It would be entirely erroneous to regard them as equivalent to instinctive activities. In the case of instinct, we are dealing with primary knowledge, inherited aptitude for activity ; acquired automatism, on the other hand, is secondary knowledge.

Finally, we may refer to a further misuse of words. Occasionally, instinctive activities on the one hand, and extreme experiential activities, and also behaviour based on insight, on the other hand, are distinguished as " unconscious " and " conscious " actions. From all that we have said above, this distinction is not allowable. For in the case of mankind, the degree of consciousness may vary greatly without any reference to the relative part played by instinctive and experiential elements in certain activities. And in the case of animals, the distinction between conscious and unconscious activities is ruled out entirely, since we know nothing whatever concerning their consciousness.

"Inborn ideas" do not exist in man. He brings into the world the aptitude for acquiring in a continually increasing degree, in the course of his individual development, concepts and abstractions ; a definite morality or a definite idea of God are no more born in him than are, for example, the concepts chair, tree, horse. He simply possesses the aptitude for acquiring such concepts relating to his environmental conditions as are brought to him by his fellow-men. He further possesses the aptitude for absorbing the moral and religious standards which are valid in his environment. Or as Jung expresses it somewhat differently : "Morality is not forced upon us from outside, we have it in ourselves a priori—not the special law and the single rule, but morality as such." If mankind possessed inborn ideas, they would be matters of highly specialized primary knowledge—a primary knowledge such as the spider, for example, would possess concerning her web, if she were conscious to the same degree, and in the same manner, as man.

Human concepts and ideas are based upon primordial aptitudes for reaction, which are also shared by animals. A large object moving quickly, an approaching beast of prey, will cause many animals to take flight or assume a defensive position ; it is on this basis that man has developed the concept of "enemy". A young chicken does not yet know the difference between what is edible and what is not ; at first it pecks at every small object, at an inkblot on the ground, and at its own toes. It only gradually learns to distinguish between what is food and what is not. On such a basis as this, man has built up the abstraction " food ". We owe to the psychiatrist Sommer the following important observation. In the case of mankind, we have cases of medium feeble-mindedness, in which abstract concepts are completely absent ; nevertheless a patient of this kind possesses a direct understanding for the things in his environment, a certain practical sense, which enables him to carry out, for example, all sorts of household duties. Sommer concludes that understanding —and insight—must be possible in the absence of abstract concepts. This is of importance in the present connection.

Behaviour based on insight, that is to say the instantaneous grasp even of an entirely new situation, has been observed in the case of a number of the highest vertebrates. Among these we have the investigation of W. Koehler and Kohts, on chimpanzees, Yerkes on gorillas, Bierens de Haan on one of the lower apes (*Cebus*), and Hertz on ravens. All these investigations were carried out with the strictest method and accompanied by critical examination of the results. We may hope that investigations of this kind will be continued, especially with reference to such animals as dogs and parrots. In this connection it is of importance always to bear in mind that the various species of animals live each in a specific " surrounding world " (in von Uexküll's sense), and therefore that human things are quite different from dog things or parrot things. Hence we never do full justice to a dog when we require it to open doors or learn to choose different colours, and then deduce its capacities from such tests. On the contrary, it is necessary to set it problems which actually belong to the dog world, to a dog situation. The corresponding case is given when pigeons, for example, are caused to run in a maze ; an experiment of this kind can never enable us to find out all the possibilities hidden in this animal. A maze has a much closer correspondence with the environment of rats or mice, and it is quite clear how different rodents and pigeons must be from one another by reason of the completely different kind of organization of their particular environmental world.

Lovers of animals are very fond of discussing the question as to whether, or how far, animals exhibit behaviour based on insight ; particularly, of course, their own animals. The lover of animals generally tends to overestimate their powers ; he looks upon inherited aptitude as insight, but his worst mistake of all is to humanize in a naïve way animal behaviour, and to overlook the fact that the surrounding worlds of his dog, his cat, and his canary, are quite different from his own.

A special form of behaviour based on insight, the use and construction of tools, is met with in apes. The chimpanzee is capable of turning a stick into an instrument for acquiring a fruit lying outside the bars of his cage. W. Koehler has observed that some of the animals kept by him were able to push one bamboo into the end of another one, or even to add to this a third, when one stick alone was too short for their purpose ; if the ends of the sticks did not fit one another at first, they were gnawed by the teeth until it was possible to fit them together. Two or three boxes were piled one on the top of another, in order to reach a fruit attached to the roof of the cage.

If the fruit was outside the cage and beyond reach, Koehler observed chimpanzees, and Yerkes gorillas, to throw all sorts of objects, even straw, for example, in its direction, and thus set up a connection, no matter how useless, between themselves and the goal. On account of the insuperable external difficulties, the apes' problem, that of reaching the fruit, could not be solved ; and not only for the observer, but also obviously for the animal, the throwing of objects towards the fruit was merely a substitute action and not a solution ; this could be deduced from the animal's whole behaviour—or in the sense of our present mode of expression : it could be understood sympathetically.

" Tool " is a quite general term for an object external to the body, and used by man or animal in addition to their own organs for carrying out any activity. According to this definition, the weaver ants living in Ceylon also exhibit the use of tools. These animals build nests in trees by a number of workers each seizing a larva of their own nests, and sticking the leaves, laid together by other workers, by means of the secretion of the larvæ. The larva may thus also be described as a tool, for it is something external to the worker's body, which it uses in addition to its own organs for spinning. This form of the use of tools is, however, something quite different from that of the apes. For in the case of the ants, we are dealing with an inherited aptitude for activity, with primary knowledge, born in every worker ; there can be no question of activity based upon insight in this case. But in the use of tools and in the construction of tools by apes, insight plays a part ; for these forms of activity are not inborn, but may arise spontaneously in a suitable situation as individual variations in behaviour.

CHAPTER X

Animal sociology.—Superindividual wholes : marriage, family, society, in man and animals.

WE said in an earlier chapter (VII) that mating, family, and society should, in the case of animals, be regarded as superindividual wholes. Obviously, the fiction of a whole can be extended to cover other cases in the organic world, according to the purpose in hand. For example, the totality of plants found in a definite limited space may be described as a whole, for between the single individuals of the same and different species living along-side one another, the most various reciprocal relations exist ; and these relations are not solely in the form of mutual competition, but may also involve exchange of material and hence be regarded as of mutual advantage (see Zimmermann). The botanist calls such communities of plants, in which one individual is dependent upon another and stands or falls with it, associations. It is a problem for plant sociology to investigate all the relation-ships occurring between plants. We are also able to take into consideration the animals which inhabit a certain locality, together with the plants ; then again we may speak of wholes, for on the one hand animal life without plants would be impossible, and on the other hand, the plants are influenced in the most various ways by the presence of the animals. Wholes of this kind are called *biocoenoses* ; according to the nature of the soil, climate, and other external factors, they are entirely different in their composition. A pond, a section of river, a mountain range, and so on, all possess their characteristic biocoenoses; the investigation of biocoenoses is called biocoenotics.

In the present connection, however, we will limit the concept of superindividual wholes to animal mating, animal families and animal societies.

These wholes are the problem of animal sociology (see my book with this title, published in 1925). The three forms we have mentioned of animal association deserve special mention here because they take effect simply as the result of factors which operate in the individuals concerned from within. Monogamic animal mating for example, is the name given to the phenomenon that one male and one female unite and live together for a longer or shorter time; in the case of many birds, the two partners thus united remain so for life, that is to say, the mating does not cease at the end of the pairing season, but persists over the period of sexual rest; this happens in the case of ravens, parrots, birds of prey, etc. It is not external compulsion that keeps the animals together. For what in all the world could lead the two partners to remain together not only during the sexual period but also during the asexual, if not their own instinct to set up such a union; the instinct for monogamic mating?

The same is true for the animal family and animal society. No external power could compel a pair of birds to take care of, to guide, and to defend their young; on the contrary, the drive to carry out all these functions acts upon the two animals from within them, and quite directly. The parental instinct of the parents corresponds to the instinct of the young to attach themselves; the drives possessed by the single individual thus lead to the animal family becoming a superindividual whole; these drives may be summarized as the instinct to form families, which exhibits itself in the case of the individual members, father, mother, and young, each in a specific manner. There likewise exists an instinct for social aggregation, which in the case of fish, birds, and mammals, for example, attaches the individual animal to the flock or herd. And this instinct causes the individual to become restless and even to waste away, when it is separated from all connection with its own kind.

Mating, family, and society of animals may be summed under the term " true societies ". We must distinguish them sharply from those chance aggregations which are the result, not of an inward instinct, but of some external factor. Writers term them *associations* as contrasted with *societies*, and hitherto I have followed this terminology. But it has led to many difficulties, above all because in plant sociology, an *association* is the term given to a number of individuals connected with one another physiologically in the closest possible manner, whereas in animal sociology, the term association has hitherto been used to describe a collection of animals brought together in one place by some external factor or other, and remaining there for a longer or shorter time without any relation to one another. It appears to me, therefore, desirable no longer to call such chance collections of animals associations, but to give them a new designation, and I propose to apply the term "conglobation" to them.

Collections of insects coming together at night around a lamp are conglobations. A single individual does not come there to associate with the other animals, but is attracted by the external factor alone, the light; and this attracts each animal without any reference to the others. Other conglobations are collections of flies and other insects on a piece of putrid meat, of green-fly on a twig, of cattle around a watering-place. It is therefore always an external factor which brings the animals together at the place in question, and they never come together there on account of the other animals. It is at first only a conglobation which results when we bring higher animals, for example birds or apes, together in a cage, or when children are collected in a school class, recruits in a squad, travellers in a railway carriage, as chance brings it about.

Whether continued existence of animals in a conglobation results in the development of a society depends upon the organization of the particular species. There are animals which are entirely incapable of entering into any kind of relationship with other individuals, or at the most those of attack and defence, and now and then the sexual act. Such animals we may call *asocietary*. In their case, every individual lives for himself, without any reference to whether it is alone or in the neighbourhood of others of its species. The lower animals, beginning with the protozoa, are throughout asocietary, and it is only in the highest animals that we find species, the members of which can form relations with one another.

H

Such species we called *societary*. Among invertebrates (molluscs) we may mention the cuttlefish (cephalopods), among the insects those that live in " states " (bees, ants, and termites), and finally among the vertebrates we have particularly birds and mammals. But even in the latter classes there are asocietary species, for example the cuckoo and the marmot.

The use of the designations societary and asocietary enables us to avoid the words *social* and *asocial*. Hitherto it was common to speak of social insects and social animals, and of social relationships between individual animals ; it was then frequently necessary to deal with the double meaning of the word social. For in its human application this term has two senses, namely one free from any reference to value, in which it merely states the presence of some kind of relationship between different persons ; and on the other hand one implying value, in which the different forms of relationship are divided morally into higher and lower. On account of this double meaning, the word social has proved unsuitable for animal psychology.

If asocietary animals are brought together at one place, the conglobation remains such, however long it exists. This can be easily shown by bringing, for example protozoa, flies, or any kind of worms together in a vessel. If, on the other hand, we are dealing with societary animals or human beings, which are of course societary by nature, the most various relations soon arise between the individuals concerned ; the conglobation thus becomes a society. We can observe this at once when a number of fowls or other birds, or apes, are brought together in a cage. In the same way, men and women brought together by chance soon set up innumerable bonds of relationship, and if sufficient time is allowed, the single individuals develop into a society.

I have already said that it is a task for animal sociology to deal with animal mating, animal family, and animal society. Occasionally the question is raised whether it is permissible to speak of such a thing as animal sociology. This objection has been raised by professional sociologists of a philosophic type of mind. It appears to me that this view is based—to put it crudely—upon an overestimate of mankind and an underestimate of animals. It was supposed that the institutions of human marriage, family, and society had come about by rational thought and resulting agreement of opinion. But if this latter idea is pursued to its logical conclusion, marriage, family, and society in mankind actually appear as business or economic undertakings. This leaves out of account altogether the completely irrational element which drives the individual human being at a given time to unite with another, to found a family, to take care of the progeny in the most self-denying manner, and also to unite with other human beings to form a society.

The objection can be made that marriage, family, and society appear in the most varied possible forms in different races and in different sections of society, and that in marriage we have, along with monogamy, polygyny, and as a rarer variation, polyandry; hence it may be said that a common denominator cannot be found. Whoever argues in this way overlooks the fact that behind all these phenomena there is the primary drive to form marital, family, and social connections, and to fulfil the demands resulting from such connections. This societary drive is—like most other drives in human beings also—very plastic, and thus may find expression in the various forms according to the environment into which the individual person is born. But it must be always present as a foundation, since otherwise marriages, families, and societies, would never come into existence in any form at all. When in a given person the societary instinct is ill-developed, whether as regards marriage, family, or society, the most severe conflicts are inevitable and it is generally not the case that the person in question fails in only one of these three respects, but equally in all of them. If, therefore, I were asked : " Are we dealing in human marriage with a business arrangement, or with a mystery ? ", I would answer, " Rather with the latter " ; for it appears to me that the irrational element is far more concerned in marriage than the pure question of mutual arrangement. The same is obviously true of family and society.

We have to imagine that in the far distant epoch when man grew up psychically beyond the animal world and became what he is today, marriage, family and society already existed, and when man then began to reflect about himself, all he could do was to sanction these already existing institutions by rational considerations formed afterwards.

We will now return to the question whether it is permissible to speak of animal sociology. We see that in many animals, a single male mates with a single female and this connection may last their lifetime ; such indi-

vidual association of the two animals with one another
I call monogamic animal mating. We have here the same
drive which leads a pair of human beings to remain
together for their lifetime for better or for worse. Hence
in man and animals, monogamic mating rests upon the
same basis; only in the case of human beings, their
much wider psychical development allows them to develop
the relationship between the two partners to a much
more differentiated degree. When in animals a male
collects several females around him—just as in many
races a man may marry several wives—we may call
this polygynic animal mating. While in some species of
animals the instinct for monogamic connection is characteristic, in others we have an instinct for polygynic
alliances.

Monogamic or polygynic mating of animals lasts either
during a reproductive period only, when we may call it
short period or seasonal mating; or the individuals in
question remain associated for a longer period and even
for life, and this we may term permanent mating. The
following distinction is also of importance. When the
individuals which have mated separate from their fellows
of the same species, we may speak of solitary mating;
we speak of societary mating, on the other hand, when
the mates live together with others in flocks or herds.
Polyandry is rare in the animal kingdom; when it occurs.
it is always connected with the female sex being consider-
ably large physically than the male.

So far, nine different categories of animal mating have
been distinguished.

(a) Polyandric, solitary, seasonal mating. Polyandry

occurs only in the case of certain invertebrates. In the case of the sea-worm *Bonellia*, for example, up to twenty dwarf males associate with every female, and live in her proboscis ; in certain spiders, two males mount the female, and repeatedly perform the sexual act.

(*b*) Monogamic solitary seasonal mating. In many species of beetle, a single male and female remain together for a summer ; the same is true of many fishes and frogs and in these cases both parents, or one at least, may also take care of the progeny. Many birds and all beasts of prey pair monogamically afresh at the beginning of each reproductive period.

(*c*) Monogamic solitary permanent mating. This form of mating is characteristic of many birds. The pair remains together even during the sexless period. It is also found in the case of the orang-utang and probably in the various species of rhinoceros.

(*d*) Monogamic societary seasonal mating. In this category we have many birds which build their nests in colonies, for example swallows, in which the pairs may remain together only for one nesting, and change their partners for the next.

(*e*) Monogamic societary permanent mating. Strict monogamic and lifelong pairing is found in the flocks of many birds, for example certain parrots. The existence of monogamic pairing within the herd is now also proved in the case of the gorilla.

(*f*) Polygynic solitary seasonal mating. This form of mating, in which the male lives with a harem only during the reproductive season, and separate from others of its species, is found in buffaloes, elephants, many species of deer, antelopes, wild sheep, and wild goats.

(g) Polygynic solitary permanent mating. Here also the male remains together with his harem for a longer time, but likewise apart from others of his species ; examples are the domestic fowl, the fuanao, the vicuna, the primitive wild horse, the zebra, the wild ass, the kangaroo, and the macaco.

(h) Polygynic societary seasonal mating. In many species of seals, for example the American fur-seal, the male collects around him a harem for the duration of the reproductive season ; sometimes numerous males with their harems are assembled at the same place. At first furious fighting for the possession of the females occurs among the males, until a gradual mutual recognition and limitation of interests is brought about.

(i) Polygynic societary permanent mating. In the herds of many apes, for example the baboon, we can discern an organization of this character ; each adult male, of which several or even many are present in a herd, collects a harem about him. The constitution of a harem remains unchanged for a considerable time.

The animals united with one another monogamically or polygynically maintain their unions more or less faithfully; here we have both specific and individual differences. Monogamy is strictly maintained among cranes, swans, and geese ; in other species of birds, unfaithfulness occurs from time to time ; we then speak of accessory promiscuity. We must distinguish sharply between two forms of promiscuity : promiscuity as a normal thing, no mating at all occurring in the species in question ; and accessory promiscuity occurring in many species alongside mating. This latter form is, as we know, not uncommon among mankind ; but in spite of earlier statements to the contrary, promiscuity as a normal thing is known to us neither in any past nor any present-day race. Among birds and mammals we have, alongside many species in which mating regularly takes place, a few species in which mating is regularly absent ; in these, therefore, promiscuity is normal. Such species are the game-fowl, North American cattle-bird, cuckoo, bat, bison, hare, quail, and pheasant. In the case of black-cock and capercailzie, the relations of the sexes approach promiscuity.

In the case of many lower animals living in water, no individual sexual relationships whatever exist, both male and female discharging into the water their sexual secretions, the ova being thus fertilized. In many lower animals sexual union takes place, but the sexual act is repeatedly or frequently performed in a quite unordered manner, between animals of opposite sex, so that promiscuity is normal. But the further we ascend in the zoological system, the more frequent become the cases where an individual alliance of shorter or longer duration occurs between the sexual partners, whether monogamic or polygynic ; in other words mating takes place.

The animal family arises from animal mating, when the individuals in question remain together for a time. According as both parents or only one remain with the offspring, or as the offspring alone remain together for a time, we distinguish the parental family, paternal family, maternal family, offspring family.

We may describe as animal societies the shoals of fish and flocks of birds and herds of mammals; many also of the invertebrate cephalopods form shoals. Chief of all, we have the " states " of bees, ants and termites (see von Frisch and Escherich). In societies of birds and mammals, monogamic associations and families may take part, and many animal societies consist solely of individuals united by mating and by family relations. Mating of the latter kind has already been termed societary.

According to the period of duration of animal societies, they may also be divided into classes. We have temporary societies in the wandering swarms of locusts and dragon-flies. These animals are as a rule solitary, and when a number of them are found together, we are confronted with a conglobation. However, a drive to wander may suddenly arise in several individuals together; they fly away in a closed swarm, and on their way attach all members of their species to them. But sooner or later, this nomad society breaks up again. Seasonal societies are of somewhat longer duration; they remain together during a year. Many birds and mammals live together in societies only during the annual sexual rest period, whereas in the reproductive season, each monogamic or polygynic family separates from the other members of the species (the first form is found in many migratory birds, the latter in the nandoo and Indian buffalo, for example). Others live in societies for the whole year, but the structure of these varies greatly from one season of the year to another; for example, the herds of the fur-seal consist in the reproductive period of males with their harems, while in the period of sexual rest males and females live in separate herds. Permanent societies may be formed both by animals exhibiting seasonal rutting, and also by species which are permanently capable of sexual union (for example, rodents living in colonies show seasonal rutting, and are monogamic; whereas many apes are permanently sexual; the gorilla being monogamic, the baboon polygynic). Every such society, therefore, is constructed of a number of monogamic or polygynic matings, and their offspring. A peculiar form of permanent society is that of the " states " of societary insects (ants, bees, and termites).

It is always inward compulsion and inhibition, which regulate the living together of animals, in mating, families, or societies. The supreme principle is not naked force; this only plays a part when irreconcilable differences occur. In animal society there is in no sense a state of confusion, either in sexual, or in any other respect, the same being of course true of aboriginal society. Let us take as an example a flock of nesting wild or tame pigeons. These animals live monogamically, nevertheless accessory promiscuity occurs, inasmuch as the sexual partners are occasionally unfaithful. It would be a complete mistake to explain the maintenance of monogamic relations between pairs of these birds merely on the basis of general want of opportunity for unfaithfulness. For a societary organization can never be durably founded on such external chances, even an organization such as that of pigeons. The most important requisite is always the inward predisposition of the animals concerned to a definite attitude, their inherited instinctive reaction towards the external world. This is, of course, supported by many accessory factors, such as fear of the sharp beaks of other paired pigeons, intensive occupation with nest building and care of the offspring. But the primary thing is the monogamic pairing instinct.

In the foregoing, we have described the three forms of society : mating, family, and social organization, as super-individual wholes, while we are of course at liberty in other connections to set up the fiction of other super-individual wholes. We selected mating, family, and society, for the reason that they result from individual association which does not depend on chance or external compulsion, but is governed by a drive, operating from within. As members of a society, the individuals in question become as it were parts of this new whole, and their behaviour can only be understood when we take into account their relation to this whole.

CHAPTER XI

Spontaneity and attention.—Understanding and communication. —Emotion and emotional transference.—Personal familiarity.—The will to superiority.

WE have seen in earlier chapters how greatly the behaviour of animals is dependent upon internal physiological states ; for the hungry animal, a piece of food has the character of a goal, and is striven after with every available means ; after hunger is satisfied, food has lost its actuality and remains unnoticed. The same is true for all other things in the animal's world ; hence we are justified in saying that one and the same individual lives in a completely different world according to its physiological state. This rule may be immediately transferred to mankind. We must further add to this that the animal's world may change not only from within the individual ; by the addition or removal of a single thing, it may be completely altered at a stroke. For the individual grasps its outside world, not additively, but as a whole, so that every single thing in it interacts intensively with every other. The appearance of an enemy, for example, fundamentally transforms the surrounding world. Suddenly, some things lose their actuality, whereas others become of importance for avoiding or fighting the opponent. The same is true of the disappearance of food or of the sexual partner ; hitherto indifferent things are made part of the external world, if they are able to serve the restoration of the original state of affairs. A peculiar type of surrounding world is that in which the goal striven for is for the moment absent. For example, the bee, acting upon its primary knowledge, seeks flowers ; and if, when it is away from the hive, we remove the latter some distance away, it seeks it on its return in the old position.

Regarding the matter from the point of view of the final result, and in the fictional sense, we may speak in both these cases, of a " search " for a thing of the external world which is not yet perceived, without reference to whether anything corresponding thereto exists in the bee's consciousness. Other animals also search, in many cases, for a goal outside their immediate perception, whether it be one that has not yet come within the range of their sense organs, or one that has subsequently been lost by some chance or another.

The behaviour of animals is not decided alone by physiological states which the observer can directly determine, such as hunger, satisfaction, capacity for pairing, fatigue, and so on ; there is something else present in addition which we must describe as spontaneity. Activity occurring spontaneously cannot be regarded merely as something happening by a release effect ; it is therefore not a newly appearing external factor which causes the change of behaviour in such cases. The whole internal situation may lead to the gradual ripening of an impulse to exclude or relax some activity or another, so that a change in behaviour is produced without external influence.

It was a fundamental mistake of earlier authors to assume that the animal is " the slave of its surroundings " or " of its sense organs "—as it was expressed—and was thus obliged to follow every sensual stimulus. On the contrary, sense impressions are only guides to it. In certain cases of course, the intra-central attitude of an animal may be decisively influenced by an external factor, for example an enemy, or by an inward physiological factor, for example hunger or want of air. But apart from these and similar causes, an animal may act spontaneously in a manner which cannot be predicted. An animal may run away, fly, or swim up, spontaneously, that is to say, without any change in its surroundings. Whether, where, and when it lies down to rest are also decided in the first place by its spontaneity.

Hence the sense impressions which the animal is continually receiving are always followed conditionally only ; spontaneity may lead an object to suddenly assume the character of a goal, and finally likewise to lose it again. This brings us to the problem of attention. It is true that biologically important factors, such as food or enemy, may be able in many cases to attract attention. But beyond this it is spontaneity which decides in the case of animals, whether anything in their surroundings shall acquire actuality or lose it ; the direction of the attention towards any object is not a reflex process, but a higher intra-central act.

We know in the case of man that a change in the external situation may have the most varied effects, such as acceleration of the pulse, palpitation, perspiration, blushing, trembling, even hair standing on end, and the like. These physiological processes are the peculiar forms of expression of internal agitation. Along with these, we may have movements of certain groups of muscles, such

as those of the face, the arms, legs and so on. Furthermore, in the case of man, we may have tears, laughter,
whistling, or even song. All these things may take place
as simple forms of expression, for example, even in the
absence of other persons. If a second person is present,
he is able to understand the psychical situation of the
first by observing the forms of expression. This frequently
happens without the first individual having produced
these forms of expression with the object of bringing
about understanding with the second. Finally, we have
the case when forms of expression are used as a means
for effecting an understanding with a fellow-creature,
and hence with the object of mutual understanding.

We have thus defined three possibilities : 1. The form
of expression appears without its reaching or being intended to reach another person. 2. It is produced without
reference to a second person, but is nevertheless grasped
and understood by one. 3. It is intended to be understood, and to bring about mutual comprehension.

In the case of mankind movements of the larynx may
also be forms of expression, and these lead in the simplest
case to expressive sounds having no conceptual meaning.
Sounds of this kind have led to the formation of human
speech. Such a thing as conceptual speech does not exist
in the case of animals, but mutual understanding may
nevertheless be brought about between them ; only,
however, among the highest species. Many animals make
use of the tail as an organ of expression ; this is easily
observed in the case of the dog, the squirrel and others.
If any object of interest, such as a piece of food, or a
member of the same species, appears within the sphere

of observation of such an animal, its tail may exhibit lively motions while its body remains still. The intra-central excitement " flows off " in this way, it is prevented from being dammed up, as has been said. Similar dis-charge of excitement is seen in the case of a person who taps with his fingers on the table, when any other reaction is for the time unavailable. The tail wagging of animals which we have mentioned is a form of expression pro-duced without reference to other animals : but how far others are also able to grasp and take notice of it, requires further investigation. Human beings at any rate take it as a quite definite signal when a dog approaches them wagging its tail. Other forms of expression found in animals are sounds of various kinds ; the song of birds also belongs in this category. A bird may sing without a member of its own species being in the neighbourhood ; it is then a matter merely of the discharge of intra-central excitement, such as occurs in connection with the general enhancement of life phenomena at the pairing period. But the song may also serve to establish a relationship between male and female, for it may be the means of rivalry between two or more males. Many forms of expression of animals such as hissing, snarling, barking, erection of the feathers or hairs, are taken by other animals as a warning signal. In all these forms of expression we are dealing with inherited, that is, instinctive, reactions, and the alarm and recoil produced by them is also instinctive. Whether or how far experience may also take part in such defence and repulsion probably varies from case to case.

Other forms of expression are the strokes of the antennæ

which the individual ant gives to another ant ; this " tickling " transfers specific states of excitement from one animal to another, so that definite activities are incited, such as feeding, search for food, common attack, flight, etc.

Many birds and mammals emit a sound at the approach of an enemy, and this sound is taken as an alarm not only by members of the same species, but also those of other species. For example, the so-called warning cry of the jay causes all animals in the wood to start. The jay by no means cries with the intention of warning the remaining creatures in the wood ; but the expressive form of the cry is taken as an important signal. In the latter case, experience plays a decisive part. The reaction to the jay's cry is not inborn ; the animals living in the wood have learned to connect danger with this cry (a biologically indifferent stimulus has become associated to them with an unconditioned stimulus), and this secondary knowledge is then carried over from one generation to the next by the example of the parents.

Inviting sounds are to be regarded as aiding mutual understanding ; finches, for example, when passing together through the wood, make continual sounds, which serve to hold the whole flock together. Bodily movements of the most varied form may be applied to bring about mutual understanding between members of the same species ; thus every species of ape possesses sounds, lip signs, bodily gestures and movements, peculiar to it, and used in intercourse with its kind. And when an imprisoned dog howls until its master comes and frees it, there can be no doubt that this form of expression, howling, is not

I

produced merely as such, but with the object of communication with its master.

The excitement which is behind these forms of expression we call emotion. The forms of expression are often characterized as over-emphasized reactions, since there is an over-production of movement and sound. The stronger the emotion, the stronger the over-emphasis—at least this is true in the majority of cases. We have seen earlier that affective expression is often without importance as regards the relationship of the individuals to one another. In other cases, the affective expression becomes a signal for another individual, and on this basis mutual understanding may come about. An emotional storm brought about by its interaction with the surrounding world may often be of biological value to an animal, for example, when it is a matter of defending itself from an enemy or overcoming its prey; but in other cases a storm of this kind may also be a danger to the individual's life, as for example if it is led to attack an opponent too powerful for it, or if it falls into a panic.

In the case of asocietary animals, other individuals enter their surrounding world only temporarily, as enemy, prey, or sexual partner; otherwise, they remain excluded. In the case of the members of societary species, the part played by other individuals is quite different; societary animals are only capable when united to their fellow-members of the species, of developing all their inherent possibilities. Societary animals may enter into mutual relations with exhibition of strong emotion. Primary knowledge causes one animal to recognize another as a member of its own species. If one dog meets another, its whole surrounding world is changed at a single stroke, its emotional reaction brings the fellow-member of its species into the centre of attention, and causes the most various forms of expression to appear. Primary knowledge allows the young chaffinch to recognize the older male as a suitable example for learning to sing, and to set its muscles in motion in a proper manner.

Likewise on account of primary knowledge, the human child of a few months of age is able, for example, to pout its lips, and make other movements of the face when these are shown to it by an adult. Here we have between two human individuals, the child and the adult, a completely direct kind of contact ; the adult is not able to state in words " how he does it " when he pouts his lips, much less is the child able to do so ; inherited primary knowledge guides the child in imitating with its own organs an example given to it.

The child also possesses an inborn resonance for affective expression ; according to an observation by Bleuler, a boy of five months already recognized the meaning of being laughed at. In this connection, we may also remark that all animals, including the anthropoid apes, are completely and finally devoid of any understanding of laughter, which is a specifically human form of expression.

When two human individuals enter into mutual relations, not only the spoken word, but also something much more direct plays a part. Look and gesture are required to give the words the necessary relief, and often even words are unnecessary to bring about understanding and sympathy. Sympathy as well as antipathy usually arise on the basis of such direct relationship, and less as the result of a conversation. Animals, for their part, do not possess speech in any form; nevertheless the members of societary species are capable of understanding one another, and this always comes about, in absence of words, by motions and sometimes by the emission of certain sounds. In this way alone, in the case of animals, individual friendships and enmities are also set up, and the sexual partners become associated in monogamic or polygynic mating.

Geiger says that in the case of societary animals, members of the same species are directly recognized as comrades.[1] This sense of comradeship may be deepened between animals which are more closely united with one another, such as mates, parents, offspring, or members of the same herd. In the " animal friendships " frequently described as existing between members of different species, we have this sense of comradeship also existing. The same comradeship may also be set up between man and dog, or man and ape. The further removed from one another in their whole organization two species are, or in the case of man, the further the animal is removed from his own species, the less can the other individual be felt as a person, and the more it becomes an object.

In flocks of finches, the most various species are found together and recognize one another mutually, as social partners; in the herds of African big game, we find various species of antelope, and even zebra and ostrich;

[1] The German is *du-evidenz*. This is untranslatable in English. It means " obviously entitled to be addressed with the familiar thou ".

in the case of ants we have mixed colonies, where two or more species are found together. But, as we have already said, when the difference in organization is too great, a limit is set to the formation of societies made up of different species.

The emotions bring the individuals of societary species in mutual relation to one another. Emotional expression of a suitable character produces frictionless interrelation, while unsuitable emotion leads to disharmony. An emotion is transferred easily from one individual to another. This accounts for the infectious character of many activities; the barking of a dog will set all the dogs in the neighbourhood barking; one bird taking to flight may sometimes cause the whole flock to follow its example. Emotions also play a decisive part in the relationship between human beings. A completely emotionless action—as far as such a thing is possible—will scarcely lead anyone to imitate it; a statement made unemotionally possesses infinitely less power to move than one accompanied by motion.

In the higher animals, the comradeship between members of like species finds its expression in their very strong affective reaction to the specific cry of fear or warning; furthermore, it is not unusual for the sight of a dead individual of the same species to produce strong emotion. Thus it is possible to keep ravens, for example, away from a fowl-run, not only by means of a scarecrow, which imitates a human being (however crudely), but also by hanging up a dead raven.

In the mutual relationships of animals which are in a more or less friendly relationship to one another, a part is played not only by mutual help, but also by mutual injury. Here we may find the manifestation of a force to which our attention has been particularly drawn by Adler's Individual Psychology : the striving for power or superiority. Schjelderup-Ebbe has made extensive investigations concerning the order of rank which is always set up in societies of birds and mammals. One individual is always the superior and one the inferior. The greater the number of individuals forming a society, the more differentiated may such a system become. Nor is it brute force alone which decides who is to be the superior ; it may be simple arrogance, and above all a peculiar bearing, which gives an individual animal superiority from the beginning. The striving for superiority may take the most various forms. Apes often show a tendency to unexpectedly pull the tail or hair of a comrade. In Koehler's experiments, one of the chimpanzees piled two or three boxes one upon the other in order to reach some suspended food ; while he was then working on the top of this structure in a precarious position, the other unoccupied chimpanzees would sometimes creep behind his back and upset the whole erection, together with the animal, by a powerful push, and then run away at great speed. At times, it would become the fashion with Koehler's chimpanzees to throw sticks at the fowls. The fowls would either be simply attracted, or even actually fed, with bread, and then be suddenly poked violently with a stick ; this game might be played by two chimpanzees working together, one feeding the fowls and the other tormenting them.

Schjelderup-Ebbe describes in the case of the wild duck

a game of a sexual character, which depended upon the deception of several males by a female. The wild duck lives monogamously, and this union is, generally speaking, very strictly adhered to by the female. A mated female was seen to fool several unpaired males on various occasions, by flying towards them, only to fly away to safety in good time, as soon as they began to run after her.

The following case in which an individual ape, itself unquestionably inferior in position, attempted to acquire a certain superiority, is reported by Yerkes. In a cage, a younger ape was accustomed to set its comrades against one another. The animal behaved as if it had been attacked by another ape ; as soon as this resulted in the elder apes quarrelling, it ran away and observed the further course of events from a secure position.

CHAPTER XII

The human being as investigating subject, and object of investigation.

In this concluding chapter, we will once more deal with human beings. I have often had to mention them before, and I believe that we have been able to show very many traits common to man and animals. I do not of course intend to eliminate the difference between man and animals; the zoologist is perhaps of all men the most familiar—almost daily and hourly in fact—with the line of division between animals and man. But we must not forget, by reason of the differences, what they have in common; and it must be especially stressed here that man can never be completely understood as a " spiritual being "; if no account is taken of the fact that he is conditioned by, and bound to, nature, he easily becomes for the investigator a ghost and a phantom.

When we take human beings as organisms among many others, we arrive at the fact that the knowledge which they are able to collect can never have absolute, but only relative, value. As von Uexküll has shown, every animal exists in its own surrounding world as under a glass globe. The same is true of human beings; every person, indeed, has his own surrounding world, which is conditioned by his physical and psychical organization. The objects constituting this world for one person are not necessarily objects forming part of the world of another.

To make a comparison ; objects reflected in mirrors of various curvatures and colour exhibit various kinds of images, and every mirror is " right " according to its own nature.

In this book I have put forward the view that we human beings are only able to grasp the world by setting up certain fictions. I must leave it to the reader to decide whether he will follow this view or not, or will demand from science doctrines which claim to be absolute. Furthermore, this decision also is a question of the psychical structure, and of the psychical needs which spring from it. Without doubt, that person is subjectively happier who sets up a rigid system of firm opinions as absolute truth.

Concerning this notion of fictions, we may also make the following further remarks. A fiction is a construction which brings into connection with one another various kinds of processes or things in a manner which enables us to think about them. A fiction is sometimes an image which serves to make a thing more picturable. A judgment as to whether the imagined connections really exist, frequently lies entirely outside the limits of our powers. The concept of a fiction, therefore, is stated here in a somewhat different sense, than in Vaihinger's philosophy of " As If ". For this author, fictions are also " consciously false assumptions, which are either in contradiction with reality or even in contradiction with one another ". Fictions of this kind may prove to be useful in other branches of science, for instance mathematics, but are not suitable to the present connection.

But in course of this book the reader may have perhaps

noticed another mode of expression, which almost has the character of a fiction in Vaihinger's sense. I spoke frequently of the " higher " and " lower " animals. In the former class we placed those more similar to human beings than those we placed in the latter. Man describes himself as the highest form ; from the point of view of human nature, as we know it in daily life this is readily comprehensible. To be able, and compelled, to select experience appears to man as a characteristic of a high rank ; but how would the position appear from the point of view of the ant or the spider ? These animals receive at birth, in the form of primary knowledge, everything that they need in the way of powers, for the rest of their life.

As compared with so rich an inherited endowment, might not man's want of primary knowledge be actually regarded as a lower characteristic ? At the beginning of the system we place the protozoa, since they consist only of a single cell. Is it not also possible to maintain the view that those organisms are the highest in which a single cell is able to exercise all the functions of life, whereas in the case of multicellular animals, millions and milliards of cells must be combined together to produce the same effects by a division of labour ? When therefore, we have spoken here of higher and lower animals, we are simply making use of conventional expressions, which have the advantage of brevity.

I have already said that it is simply a question of psychical need which decides the fiction set up by an investigator. Nature only answers those questions which we ask her ; indeed, she only gives the observer those answers which he expects from her. The interpretation of what happens in the case of man or animals is thus a matter of the psychological structure of the observer ; the psychical quality of the individual scientist is responsible for the nature of the surrounding world which he builds up for himself ; it decides what things and processes are invested with actuality in it, and what are ignored as unimportant. Furthermore, every variety of world view can be linked with the results of our observation in nature. Thus mechanists and vitalists, for example, may actually use the same experiments to serve as " proof " of their views.

It is a strange thing that controversies such as that between vitalism and mechanism are possible at all. The defenders of these two points of view appear on the scene with a claim to absolute validity for their doctrines, and overlook the fact that they are dealing only with fictions which each is opposing to the other. Driesch, one of the most eminent vitalists of our time, is a true child of the period in which he received the directive stimulus for his life ; he is a rationalist exactly like his great opponent, the mechanist Roux. The method of thought of both is rationalist, Driesch believing that the irrational can be grasped by reason. Driesch's four proofs of vitalism will doubtless appear to a later time much the same, as today the proofs of God's existence found in older theology and philosophy appear to us.

Causality and finality are therefore nothing but two fictional aspects ; purely causal views in biology stress the strict succession of events, whereas the finalist view takes the events of the living world from the point of

view of the whole, and makes the fiction of some " end "
in the statistically determined final result.   Causality
and finality are not something read off from natural
events in the " external world ", but have been put into
it by human beings, as a result of the need for the
recognition of an order.

The causal law also, which is by the way not denied
by present-day vitalists, is also a fiction.   It cannot be
proved in the strict sense, for this would require us to
know all natural processes which have ever taken place,
are taking place, and will take place in the world.   Nevertheless, the law of causality is, on the one hand, a psychical
necessity for us, at least, in so far as non-living nature is
concerned ;   and on the other hand, we have no alternative
but to assume such a law, since otherwise all our scientific
and technical endeavours would appear meaningless from
the start.

The fact that we exist, and are just as we are, is a fact
which lies for us entirely in the irrational sphere.   We
have received a number of drives, in general of an extremely plastic character, which compel us to develop
our psychical organisation at the same rate as our
physical ;   these endeavours of ours are connected with
ideals, which were the subjects of our choice.   Let no
one say that persons exist who are devoid of ideals.   It
is true that not everyone strives after ideals approved
by society, of a humanitarian, occupational, or similar
nature ;   but there exist ideals of a very different character,
formed as the result of peculiar internal and external
situations.   Everyone has some ideal, some goal, after
which he strives openly or secretly ;   everyone must

clothe his affirmation of life in some form.   Nothing else
is allowed by the drive which operates in the individual.

Not only is the beginning and end of our existence
irrational, but also its whole course.   Those who see in
the fundamentals of human life no problem at all, are
able by the aid of the facts which have been learned by
experience, to " explain " all sorts of things rationalistic-
ally, and may even finally be led to the idea of solving
" the riddle of the universe ".   Only, they overlook the
fact that all fundamentals are assumed as existing, and
hence the real problem is entirely set aside.

Our existence cannot be understood purely from the
point of view of biological utility.   Rather do we see
everywhere irrational drives at work, which drive both
individuals and also whole groups again and again to new
plans and deeds.   Inventions are not made because
definite needs exist, which have to be satisfied, but
inversely : first we have the invention, and only later
does the possibility of practically applying it appear.
Thus the microscope, for instance, was for centuries an
instrument used by amateurs, who devoted themselves to
observing the minute without reference to practical purposes ; it was only in our day that it has become an
indispensable instrument for the physician.   The same
may be said of all other inventions.   The steamship and
the railway were rejected when first introduced.   The
telegraph and telephone were not invented because it
had been found that humanity could not get on without
them ; after decades of investigation by physicists without
any useful object, the moment came when practical
utility was seen to be possible ; but the public was com-

pletely indifferent to the first attempt to introduce the telephone. We may finally mention two inventions of most recent date; the aeroplane and airship. Here no one will maintain that they were created because it was impossible to get along without them.

At the back of everything that man undertakes we have therefore the drive which imperatively demands activity. It is true that our occupation serves the purpose of breadwinning; but this useful purpose is not in the first place decisive as regards occupational activity; much more important is the presence of the irrational drive to form something, build up something, and to carry it on continually. It is thus that business, industry, and agricultural undertakings come about, thus the general creates his army, the statesman, the writer, the scientist, do their life's work. The irrational element is particularly evident in the activity drive of the artist and of those interested in religion. Religion no more serves a purpose than does art; art is not intended to give pleasure, to elevate, to amuse, or whatever other banal purposes may be ascribed to it; it is a form of expression, in which the artist clothes his inmost experience, and here and there his work of art then meets with human beings who are able sympathetically to understand his form of expression, and feel within themselves an inward resonance to it. In this way, a work of art is able to bring about an inter-individual relationship by the transference of emotion.

It is not the accomplishment of just sufficient to carry on life, but overproduction, which has an emotional and pleasurable tone; this is true both of the occupational as well as for other spheres. Dance, games, and sport have not been invented to provide human beings with recreation, but have originated as forms of expression of the activity drive immanent in man. We are able to observe the gradual development of this drive in the case of every child ; it is manifested in new ways as the child develops from stage to stage, in learning to walk and talk, in playing, and so on. Regarded causally, the child's play appears simply conditioned by the physiological and psychological factors operating in it ; regarded finalistically—taking therefore the state of the adult as the fictional " goal "—play serves as practice for future behaviour.

In this book, we have set up the fiction that man and animal are related in nature, so that conclusions can be drawn from one to another regarding their life processes. The plants also could be drawn into this community of nature. At the same time, the world of organisms was contrasted with non-living nature, peculiar laws being assumed for the living world ; a psyche-like agent was imagined as responsible for the phenomena of life exhibited by the organism. In the present connection, it was sufficient to ascribe to each single individual such an agent ; it was not necessary to form the fiction of super-individual, or collective, psyche-like agents, which could be manifested in society. Now plants, animals, and man form an uninterrupted developmental series of forms. How far it may be advantageous to assume psyche-like agencies as responsible for this continual further development, or philogenesis, will not be discussed here ; we may only refer to the possibility.

We cannot speak of a plant psychology. We certainly set up the fiction that a psyche-like agent is behind the life phenomena of plants; but the latter are not able to execute bodily movements, such as occur in endless variety in the case of animals and man. These movements are what form the object of animal and human psychology. The observer is only able to draw psychological conclusions from the form and degree of motions which he observes; expressive movements and sounds of all kinds, as well as human speech, belong to this category.

CONCLUSION

WE may now shortly summarize the main points of what has been said.

In this book we have made use of the view that human beings are compelled to set up fictions in order to comprehend themselves and the world surrounding them. It is not given to us to attain absolute knowledge, but only that which is adapted to our sense organs and our mental organization. Furthermore, the nature and character of " knowledge " depends in the first place upon the psychical nature of the " knower ". We take as fictions all natural laws, including that of causality, the assertions of mechanism and vitalism, the doctrine of the freedom and non-freedom of the will, and so on.

In the foregoing we have made use of the fiction that life events, as opposed to processes taking place in the non-living world, follow special laws ; not, however, in the sense that life infringes physical and chemical laws, but that its special laws are built up on the latter as a foundation. It was further assumed that man and animals obey the same laws as regards their bodily and psychical processes, although they manifest themselves to us differently in their details.

Our psychical organization allows us to grasp not only ourselves, but also the surrounding world, as a whole. Only afterwards do we break up our surroundings into single things, and as regards the things individually, the whole is again present to us before the part. Likewise, in the case of our own actions, the whole is given before the parts. In order to grasp the organism and its activities, we have made use of the fiction " the wholeness of the individual " ; we assumed as super-individual wholes, both in the case of man and animals, mating, family, and society.

The observer collects statistical experience as to how certain modes of behaviour or bodily processes usually take place in man and animals ; on the basis of this knowledge, the life process appears to him under the form of the fiction that the whole determines the parts, and the end determines the means. Here the " whole " is the course of bodily development or of a certain activity, as predictable by the observer, and the " end " is the final state. In the non-living world, there is no whole and no end in the sense of the words as here employed.

We may further set up the fiction that in organisms there exists, behind the whole life process, a psyche-like agent. Our consciousness would then be that region in which this agent is able to grasp itself. The question as to the consciousness of animals is insoluble. It has also declined in importance, as recent medical deep psychology has taught us, that in the case of man, the contents of consciousness often do not determine the ultimate action.

In grasping the behaviour of a fellow-human being, we have to distinguish between the methods of " understanding " and " explaining ". The first takes place as a process of direct sympathy and comprehension, the latter depends upon experience and statistics. The physician, for example, is sometimes able to understand a neurotic, even when the latter does not understand the aim of his neurosis, and hence does not understand himself. Hence the process of understanding does not always depend upon the conscious mind of the person understood. Hence, under the fiction that man and animals are allied in nature, we may make use of the understanding and sympathetic method, along with the explanatory, in animal psychology. On the other hand, one person can understand another directly in the more comprehensive sense meant here, without necessarily being clearly and sharply conscious of his behaviour. Hence in understanding, even the actual content of the understander's consciousness does not always play the chief part.

Leaving out the question of consciousness, we have set up the fiction that the animal also grasps itself and the peculiarities of its surroundings as a whole. Direct understanding is possible between animals: the more distant the species of two animals, the more difficult is understanding. Between man and animal, mutual understanding is also possible within limits. But man is often excluded from such understanding of animal behaviour because much in the animal takes place on the basis of inherited aptitude for activity (instinct, primary knowledge), whereas man, for his part, is obliged to acquire by experience, as secondary knowledge, practically everything.

The inherited and instinctive element exceeds by far the experiential, in most cases of animal behaviour. Instinctive and experiential activity are not sharp con-

K*

trasts, but extremes of an endless series of intermediates. For many instinctive actions are not completely rigid, but in so far plastic as they are capable of individual modifications based upon experience. On the other hand, even in the case of man, every experiential action contains some element of the instinctive.

Behaviour based on insight is found, apart from man, in some of the highest vertebrates (for example, ravens and apes). In actions based on insight there is also always an instinctive component ; modern deep psychoogy has the credit for pointing out the part played by instinctive drives in human behaviour.

BIBLIOGRAPHY

ADLER, A., *The Practice and Theory of Individual Psychology*, trans. by P. Radin, London, 1924. A 4th German Edition was published in 1930.

ALVERDES, F., *Neue Bahnen in der Lehre vom Verhalten der niederen Organismen*, Berlin, 1923.

ALVERDES, F., *Social Life in the Animal World*, trans. by K. C. Creasy, London, 1927.

ALVERDES, F., "Die Frage nach der Ganzheitlichkeit in der Verhaltensweisen der Tieren," *Biologia Generalis*, Vol. 7, 1931.

BIERENS DE HAAN, J. A., "Werkzeuggebrauch und Werkzeugherstellung bei einem niederen Affen," *Zeitschrift für vergleichende Physiologie*, Vol. 13, 1930.

BLEULER, E., *Die Psychoide als Prinzip der organischen Entwicklung*, Berlin, 1925.

BUDDENBROCK, W. v., *Grundriss der vergleichenden Physiologie*, Berlin, 1928.

BUDDENBROCK, W. v., "Tropismen," in Gellhorn's *Lehrbuch der allgemeinen Physiologie*, Leipzig, 1931.

DRIESCH, H., *The Science and Philosophy of the Organism*, 2nd. Ed., London, 1929.

ESCHERICH, K., *Die Termiten oder weissen Ameisen*, Leipzig, 1909.

ESCHERICH, K., *Die Ameise*, 2nd. Ed., Brunswick, 1917.

FRISCH, K. v., *Aus dem Leben der Bienen*, Berlin, 1927.

FREUD, S., *Introductory Lectures on Psychoanalysis*, trans. by Joan Riviere, London, 1922. Later German Edition, Vienna, 1930.

GEIGER, TH., "Das Tier als geselliges Subjekt," in *Forschungen zur Völkerpsychologie und Soziologie*, Vol. 10, Leipzig, 1930.

GROOS, K., *The Play of Animals*, trans. by E. L. Baldwin, with Preface and Appendix by J. M. Baldwin, London, 1898.

HEMPELMANN, F., *Tierpsychologie vom Standpunkt des Biologen*, Leipzig, 1926.

HERTER, K., *Tierphysiologie*, Vols. 1 and 2, Berlin and Leipzig, 1927 and 1928.

HERTZ, M., " Das optische Gestaltproblem und der Tierversuch." *Verh. der Deutschen Zoologischen Gesellschaft*, Vol. 33, 1929.

JENNINGS, H. S., *Behaviour of the Lower Organisms*, New York, 1906.

JORDAN, H. J., *Allgemeine vergleichende Physiologie der Tiere*, Berlin and Leipzig, 1929.

JUNG, C. G., *Das Unbewusste im normalen und kranken Seelenleben*, 3rd Ed., Zurich, 1926.

JUNG, C. G., *Psychology of the Unconscious*, trans. by B. M. Hinkle, London, 1921.

KAFKA, G., " Tierpsychologie," in *Handbuch der vergleichende Psychologie*, Vol. 1, Munich, 1922.

KRETSCHMER, E., *Medizinische Psychologie*, 3rd Ed., Leipzig, 1926.

KRETSCHMER, E., *Physique and Character*, trans. by W. H. Sprott, London, 1925.

KOEHLER, W., *Die Physichen Gestalten in Ruhe und im stationären Zustand*, Brunswick, 1920.

KOEHLER, W., *Gestalt Psychology* (trans.), London, 1930.

KOEHLER, W., *The Mentality of Apes*, London, 1929.

KOHTS, N., *The Mind of a Chimpanzee*, Psyche Miniatures, London, 1925.

KÜHN, A., *Die Orientierung der Tiere im Raum*, Jena, 1919.

KÜHN, A., " Phototropismus und Phototaxis der Tiere," in *Handbuch der normalen und pathologischen Physiologie*, Vol. 12/1, Berlin, 1929.

LEGEWIE, H., " Organismus und Umwelt," in *Forschungen zur Völkerpsychologie und Soziologie*, Vol. 10, Leipzig, 1931.

LOEB, J., *Forced Movements, Tropisms, and Animal Conduct*, Philadelphia and London, 1918.

MAST, S., *Light and the Behaviour of Animals*, New York, 1911.

ROUX, W., " Das Wesen des Lebens," in *Kultur der Gegenwart*, Part III, Section IV, Vol. 1, Leipzig and Berlin, 1915.

SCHJELDERUP-EBBE, TH., " Die Despotie im sozialen Leben der Vögel," in *Forschungen zur Völkerpsychologie und Soziologie*, Vol. 10, Leipzig, 1931.

SOMMER, R., *Tierpsychologie*, Leipzig, 1926.

STEKEL, W., *Psychoanalysis and Suggestion Therapy, their technique*, *etc.*, trans. by J. S. Van Teslaar, London, 1923.

UEXKÜLL, J. v., *Umwelt und Innenwelt der Tiere*, 2nd Ed., Berlin, 1921.

UEXKÜLL, J. v., *Theoretical Biology*, trans. by D. L. Mackinnon, London, 1926.

VAIHINGER, H., *The Philosophy of ' As If '*, translated by C. K. Ogden, London, 1924.

WERTHEIMER, M., *Drei Abhandlungen zur Gestalttheorie*, Berlin, 1925.

YERKES, R. M. and A. W., *The Great Apes*, New Haven, 1929.

ZIMMERMANN, W., " Pflanzensoziologie," in *Forschungen zur Völkerpsychologie und Soziologie*, Vol. 10, Leipzig, 1931.

INDEX

153